Health Promotion - Principles and Approaches

Edited by Bishan Swarup Garg

Published in London, United Kingdom

Health Promotion - Principles and Approaches
http://dx.doi.org/10.5772/intechopen.107637
Edited by Bishan Swarup Garg

Contributors
Annamária Juhász, Péter Habil Fritz, Brandon S. Shaw, Ina Shaw, Musa L. Mathunjwa, Esther Seloilwe, Kebope Mongie Kealeboga, Joyce Khutjwe, Lesedi Mosebetsi, Tebogo Mamalelala, Tanji Hoshi, Rajshri Roy, Jessica Malloy, Arild Berg, Jorunn Marie Andersen, Safora Johansen, Anne Lund, Michael Alexander Riegler, Alf Trojan, Christian Lorentz, Stefan Nickel

First published in London, United Kingdom, 2023 by IntechOpen
IntechOpen is the global imprint of INTECHOPEN LIMITED, registered in England and Wales, registration number: 11086078, 5 Princes Gate Court, London, SW7 2QJ, United Kingdom

British Library Cataloguing-in-Publication Data
A catalogue record for this book is available from the British Library

Additional hard and PDF copies can be obtained from orders@intechopen.com

Health Promotion - Principles and Approaches
Edited by Bishan Swarup Garg
p. cm.
Print ISBN 978-1-83768-428-1
Online ISBN 978-1-83768-450-2
eBook (PDF) ISBN 978-1-83768-451-9

Meet the editor

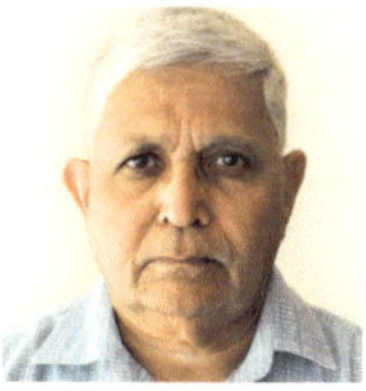

Dr. Bishan S Garg, MD, Ph.D., is secretary of the Kasturba Health Society, India, and previous dean of the Mahatma Gandhi Institute of Medical Sciences (MGIMS), India. He is an Emeritus Professor in the Department of Community Medicine and the director of the Dr. Sushila Nayar School of Public Health, MGIMS. He is also the director of the WHO Collaborating Center for Research and Training in Community-Based Maternal, Newborn and Child Health. He received the Best Teacher Award from the Maharashtra University of Health Sciences, India, in 2005 in recognition of his academic achievements and contributions. He completed numerous fellowships, including a Commonwealth Medical Fellowship at the Liverpool School of Tropical Medicine, UK, a fellowship from the National Academy of Medical Sciences (NAMS), fellowship of Indian Association of Preventive and Social Medicine (IAPSM), fellowship of Indian Public Health Association, and fellowship of Indian Society for Malaria and Other Communicable Diseases. He was also bestowed with the Sir Shriram Memorial Award by NAMS in 2008, a Dhanwantari Oration in 2004, a Dr. Harcharan Singh Oration in 2007 from the IAPSM, and an Indian Epidemiology Association Oration in 2014. He has written four books, five book chapters, and twenty-two monographs on priority public health issues. He has also published more than 180 research papers in international and national journals. He was president of IAPSM in 2002. Dr. Garg has been awarded more than eighty research projects by various funding organizations. He has served as a consultant to WHO, UNICEF, the Department for International Development (DFID), and various other international and national agencies on issues of public health concern.

Contents

Preface

"In a well-ordered society the citizens know and observe the laws of health and hygiene. It is established beyond doubt that ignorance and neglect of the laws of health and hygiene are responsible for the majority of diseases to which mankind is heir."

Mahatma Gandhi

The 21st century has witnessed significant progress in the field of health. In spite of the COVID pandemic, remarkable achievements have been made in reducing the number of people living in poverty, increasing primary school enrolment, and reducing child and maternal mortality. The number of new malaria cases and HIV infection have also declined and a considerable number of people worldwide now have access to safe drinking water and basic sanitation. However, inequity in every part of the world still exists. At the same time, lifestyle disorders like hypertension, diabetes, cancer, and obesity have increased considerably not only in the developed world but also in developing countries, affecting all segments of society, both poor and rich as well as urban and rural areas. In this scenario, health promotion, including teaching people about the health benefits of consuming a balanced diet, engaging in physical activities, and changing behaviors to minimize anxiety, stress, depression, and other mental health issues, is even more important.

This book presents the basics of and approaches to health promotion and disease prevention. It is organized into two sections. Section 1, "Basics of Health Promotion", includes three chapters. Chapter 1 emphasizes the benefits of physical activity to improve health and prevent diseases like cardiovascular diseases, obesity, diabetes, musculoskeletal problems, stress, anxiety, and depression in all populations and ages. Chapter 2 describes a social innovation-based pilot project in health promotion. The project is based on a model of holistic health consciousness and responsibility involving the participation of community residents and local actors in a health promotion program. Chapter 3 discusses a social innovation of health promotion centers that were established with natural ingredients and modern technological tools providing personalized services for primary and secondary prevention and population-based health promotion. It formulated and implemented a developmental concept based on research findings, built on it with educational implementation, and integrated communication for audiences. Using a holistic approach (physical–spiritual–mental–social), the program increased the number of healthy years of life and led to a positive experience for the participants and thus may be a promising model for other communities.

Section 2, "Approaches to Health Promotion", includes four chapters. Chapter 4 demonstrates the causal relationship between healthy life expectancy, socioeconomic status, dietary habits, lifestyle habits, and three health factors. As described by the World Health Organization (WHO), the study might be of great importance for elderly individuals, emphasizing the importance of income maintenance rather than focusing on diet and lifestyle improvements. Chapter 5 highlights that collaboration between health services and health-promoting environments may be influenced by patients, health professionals, and other stakeholders based on Antonovsky's concept of salutogenesis of promotion of a sense of coherence and the feeling of meaningfulness and people's ability to influence their own situation. An interdisciplinary understanding of a sense of coherence as described in this study can strengthen collaboration in health and technology. The results of the case study from Norway present the potential for replication of the approach in different settings in other countries. Chapter 6 describes how social media has transformed people's communication and has emerged as a powerful tool in health promotion and health policy. The chapter shares success stories from New Zealand and demonstrates that social media can also be a powerful platform for advocacy and activism to raise awareness about health-related issues, organize events and campaigns, and mobilize support for policy advocacy. Chapter 7 examines health promotion and its usefulness in preventing diseases in Botswana and concludes that health promotion has enabled people to exert control over their health and cultivate a positive health concept through participation and involvement.

This book provides useful information about the principles of health promotion and its applications in different settings. I am thankful to IntechOpen for providing me with the opportunity to edit this book. My special thanks to Publishing Process Manager Mr. Dominik Samardzija for his valuable support.

Dr. Bishan Swarup Garg MD, Ph.D., FAMS
Emeritus Professor of Community Medicine,
Mahatma Gandhi Institute of Medical Sciences,
Wardha, Maharashtra, India

Secretary,
Kasturba Health Society,
Wardha, Maharashtra, India

Section 1

Basics of Health Promotion

Chapter 1

Physical Activity and Health Promotion: A Public Health Imperative

Ina Shaw, Musa L. Mathunjwa and Brandon S. Shaw

Abstract

Continuing epidemiological and clinical studies have accumulated evidence that appropriate regular physical activity (PA) results in significant health benefits and can even prevent and treat many diseases like cardiovascular diseases, obesity, diabetes, musculoskeletal problems, stress, anxiety, and depression. These benefits are universal to all populations and age groups making physical activity a critical component in reducing many of the leading causes of global mortality. Additional benefits have also been found to follow an expanding quantity and quality of PA through the proper manipulation of the exercise design (i.e., frequency, intensity, duration, and mode). Global health benefits are achievable through physical activity, but this requires competent health professionals able to prescribe appropriate physical activity to their clients, patients, and communities to ensure engagement in increasing their PA levels and thus contribute to their own well-being and the prevention of the main non-communicable chronic diseases (NCDs).

Keywords: epidemiology, exercise, disease prevention, intervention, measurement, surveillance, wellbeing, wellness

1. Introduction

Physical activity can be described as any deliberate bodily movement generated by the skeletal muscles requiring bioenergetics [1]. Physical activity can encompass all activities, at any intensity and includes both exercise and incidental (i.e., not planned, structured, repetitive, or purposeful) activity integrated into daily routine [2]. However, global physical activity guidelines and recommendations exist based on the amount of exercise required to reap the health benefits of physical activity. One such guideline advises that individuals aged 18 years and older should accumulate 150 minutes of moderate-intensity activity per week, or equivalent [3].

Regular physical activity involvement has been linked with a significant decrease in the risk for premature mortality. It has similarly been found to decrease the risks of more than 25 chronic conditions [4, 5]. Specifically, research has demonstrated substantial evidence that regular physical activity is related to a reduced risk for all-cause mortality and numerous chronic conditions such as cardiovascular disease, ischemic heart disease, and ischemic stroke, type 2 diabetes, gestational diabetes, hypertension, breast cancer, colon cancer and gallstone disease [6]. Problematically, this guideline is overly simplistic because certain physical activity modalities have been demonstrated to promote health, contribute to disease prevention and rehabilitation in different ways and through different mechanisms.

In this regard, aerobic physical activity modalities have unequivocally been found to have significant cardiorespiratory benefits and reduce the incidence of and mortality from cardiovascular and metabolic diseases from multiple mechanisms including inter alia, anti-ischemic, anti-atherosclerotic, anti-thrombotic, and anti-arrhythmic, effects in addition to its psychological health benefits encompassing reductions in anxiety, depression, and stress [7]. In turn, resistance activities have been found to exert its own plethora of health-promoting and disease prevention benefits such as reducing low back pain, arthritic discomfort, while promoting functional independence and status, and mobility [8, 9]. Resistance activities have also been demonstrated to be the most superior exercise modality to increase metabolic rate, lean body mass and bone mineral density [9]. It is for this reason that resistance activities are now endorsed for inclusion into an all-inclusive physical activity programme by various global health organisations, including the American College of Sports Medicine, American Heart Association, and the American Association of Cardiovascular and Cardiopulmonary Rehabilitation and Surgeon General's Office [10]. As such, any physical activity programme aimed at improving health and preventing disease should focus on including regular aerobic and muscular fitness activities, as well as reducing time sedentary behaviour.

1.1 The pandemic of physical inactivity

Globally, one in four adults (25%) do not meet these globally recommended levels of physical activity. This figure is even more alarming in the global adolescent population where more than 80% of adolescents have been found to be insufficiently physically active [3]. In the United Kingdom (UK), physical inactivity is linked to one in six deaths and costs the UK £7.4 billion annually. Unfortunately, the UK population is proposed to be approximately 20% less active than in the 1960s with projections that the population will be 35% less active by 2030 [11].

2. Consequences of physical inactivity

A lack of sufficient daily physical activity is an underappreciated primary cause of most chronic conditions with vast evidence demonstrating that physical inactivity results in a plethora of both physical and mental ill health conditions. Such physical health conditions include obesity, diabetes, certain types of cancer, and cardiovascular diseases [6, 12]. Some of the mental ill health conditions include declines in memory, and increases in anxiety, and depression [13].

3. Benefits of physical activity

Overwhelming scientific data has accumulated that demonstrates the significant health benefits linked to regular physical activity [11]. Participants of regular physical activity experience a multitude of physical, psychological, and social benefits.

Physiologically, regular physical activity can improve all systems of the body leading to inter alia improved cardiorespiratory fitness, muscular fitness (including muscular strength and endurance), body composition, flexibility, and balance [14, 15]. Physical activity has even demonstrated to have a positive influence on dietary behaviour [16]. However, health is determined by both the lack of disease and an individual's resistance to pathogenic factors [17]. In this area, physical activity has demonstrated its effectiveness at reducing an individual's risk of developing numerous chronic conditions and diseases [6]. In fact, individuals who engage in insufficient physical activity have a 20–30% increased risk of death compared to individuals who are sufficiently active [3].

Research has also indicated the positive impact on several areas of an individual's psychology. In this regard, studies have been found to demonstrate that physical activity has confirmed beneficial effects on sleep [18], independent function [19], overall mood [18], cognition [20], self-esteem [21], stress [22], and depression [23]. While regular physical activity has demonstrated these effects in both clinical and non-clinical settings, a greater magnitude of improvements has been demonstrated in a clinical environment in those patients with manifest mental illness [24]. It is for this reason that physical activity has a significant role in the management of mental health conditions, such as depression and anxiety [24]. However, it must be noted that studies have shown that in addition to its beneficial effects, excessive physical activity may lead to overtraining and impair mental health specifically generating psychological symptoms that mimic depression [24].

3.1 Mechanism of effect of physical activity and physical health

The improvement of health and prevention of disease depends on the mechanisms of general adaptation and enhanced homeostatic regulation and [25]. In this regard, there are several changes which are essential both for increasing adaptivity and for increased human performance [26]. Such changes that improve health and prevent disease include improvements in immunoactivities such as central nervous regulation and function, increased endocrine system function, higher insulin sensitivity, improvement in the capacity of the oxygen transport system, improvements in oxygen intake, delivery, and usage, increases in metabolic function, increased energy potential, and increases in functional stability [25, 26]. Further, physical activity has direct positive influences on the cardiovascular system including lower systemic blood pressure, increased availability of vasodilatory mediators such as nitric oxide, enhanced myocardial contractility, improved lipoprotein metabolism, enhanced ageing-related calcium distribution leading to an enhanced antisclerotic effect of physical activity, improved diaphragm and respiratory muscle strength increasing air flow through the lungs, reduction of respiratory mucous, and an increase oxygen levels [27–29].

3.2 Mechanism of effect of physical activity and mental health

Mental disorders are a major public health concern. There are numerous hypotheses proposing the mechanism of the effect of physical activity on mental health [24]. Despite the limited research on the mechanistic effects of physical activity on mental health it is thought that improvements in mental health arise from a combination of both psychological and physiological mechanisms, comprising endorphins, neurotransmitters, and the hypothalamic-pituitary-adrenal axis, and via the thermogenic hypothesis [30].

A possible psychological mechanism by which physical activity may improve mental health is related to the distraction hypothesis. Distraction is proposed to move individuals away and distract them from stressful stimuli and into physical activity [31]. Further, many individuals find physical activity to be psychologically and physically challenging. By overcoming such challenges through it is proposed that an individual's self-efficacy improves, leading to an improved self-confidence and mood [31].

Physiologically, the most well-known mechanism by which physical activity affects mental health is through endorphins, which are endogenous opioids. Specifically, physical activity has been demonstrated to positively impact mental well-being, mood, and common mental disorders and their symptoms through the enhanced release of beta endorphins [31]. It is also thought that physical activity affects mental health through brain monoamines, such as dopamine, norepinephrine, and serotonin, which are the three foremost monoamine neurotransmitters demonstrated to be impacted upon by physical activity [32]. However, different physical activity, and specifically the intensities at which they are performed, may cause varied amounts of feedback in the hypothalamus-pituitary gland-adrenal gland axis and should be taken into consideration when developing physical activity public health interventions for mental health [32]. Another proposed physiological mechanism by which physical activity may positively influence mood is through thermogenesis or the production of the body because of an increased energy production required for the physical activity. It is this thermogenesis, that like a warm bath, is proposed to result in relaxation and a better mood [31].

4. Barriers to physical activity

Thanks to sustained global and national efforts, it is increasingly rare that individuals do not know that physical activity has demonstrable benefits for both physical and mental health. However, despite knowing the multitude of benefits associated with regular physical activity, many individuals still experience barriers preventing them from engaging in physical activity. Barriers can be recognised as either physical, psychological, or socio-ecological.

Identifying the barriers and motivators contribute toward the development of specific physical activity health promotion interventions [33]. Recent studies have suggested that barriers prohibiting engagement in physical activity in adults relate mainly to environmental factors and resources, while motivators facilitating engagement in physical activity relate to health benefits, social influences, reinforcement, and assistance in managing change [33].

As such, physical activity public health interventions should focus on overcoming deficiencies in environmental factors and resources. This could be achieved by for example presenting physical activities in the community, effectively reducing environmental factors, such as the extreme cold weather conditions and limiting street environment indicators [34]. Further, physical activity public health interventions could mitigate the effect of resources by making use of existing resources in the community (i.e., community centers for delivery of interventions) and design appropriate physical activity interventions for use in these facilities based on their low supervisory requirements and cost implications [35]. To ensure the effectiveness of the community- and population wide interventions based on motivating factors, physical activity interventions could promote and objectively monitor the health benefits associated with the physical activity intervention. With regards to social influences and reinforcement, physical activity interventions should make use of activities such as group, rather than individual, interventions.

5. Physical activity as a public health intervention

Public health covers both illness prevention and promotion of personal wellbeing. Today's public health requires an inter- and multi-disciplinary team of public health workers that can implement a variety of preventive and/or responsive interventions, including epidemiology, outreach, screening, health teaching, social marketing, and policy development. Due to physical activities ability to contribute to numerous spheres of public health, it has become an integral component of public health systems [36, 37].

Research in the physical activity adherence has resulted in the recognition of several methods to influence an uptake of physical activity at the individual level [38]. However, the considerable prevalence of inactivity across most sectors of the global population necessitates higher-level approaches to physical activity promotion that include environmental, organisational, and policy-level strategies.

Physical activity provides an ideal population-wide public health intervention due to it efficacy and its low-cost ideally suited to the limited resource environment public health decision makers frequently find themselves in [39]. In this regard, many physical activity interventions require little/no equipment, require minimal supervision (in those without high risk), and can be delivered in community settings. Further, many health professionals such as physiotherapists, Biokineticists, and exercise physiologists are already serving in communities and at a population level in many countries, including low- and middle-income countries (LMICs) [40]. Where communities and countries exist that do not have such professionals specifically trained in physical activity, there is opportunity for roles and training for physical activity awareness and prescription to be offered to other healthcare professionals, such as public health practitioners, and nurses, already well placed in communities, at schools, and at a population level.

It is important to understand how physical activity affects the whole ecology. In this regard, physical inactivity and its associated morbidity and mortality affects the home, school, and workplace. It is this pervasive importance that should ensure that physical activity considerations be utilised in local strategy, policy and planning and enhancements to the built or natural physical environment to improve public spaces, workplaces, and schools to boost and provide individuals of all sectors, ages, and abilities access to physical activity.

Physical activity is imperative at a local community level due to its significant impact on physical and mental wellbeing. Determining methods for individuals in communities to enjoy physical activity can encourage regular physical activity participation. This can be achieved by prioritising pedestrians, cyclists and individuals who utilise public transport, involving community members in creating and managing public spaces [41].

Limited evidence exists to demonstrate the most appropriate methods to enhance physical activity in young children, especially considering declining school participation in sports and removal of physical education programmes [42]. However, the inclusion of parents in public health initiatives to perform parental goal setting with their children regarding physical activity have been found to be successful. Further, parental monitoring, having physical activity training providers, and encouraging healthy role-modelling in schools could increase children's levels of physical activity and could lead to healthier familial and school environments. This increase in physical activity is especially important in that being active in childhood has unequivocally been shown to encourage physical activity participation into adulthood [41].

The workplace presents an ideal setting to promote and deliver physical activity initiatives. This is because physical activity in the workplace provides the opportunity to overcome one of the most common barriers to regular physical activity namely a 'lack of time'. Workplace physical activity programmes also provide access to physical activity to a large portion of society [43]. Apart from the long-term physical and mental health benefits associated with physical activity, when physical activity is promoted in the workplace it has been shown to decrease conditions that contribute to absenteeism associated with illness, improve productivity and staff retention, decrease the costs for employers, and increase loyalty [41].

6. The way forward in addressing the pandemic of physical inactivity

Although physical activity guidelines have evolved considerably over the las few decades, due to ever-increasing physical inactivity, many public health organisations have attempted to develop physical activity intervention programmes that are more palatable to the sedentary and have recommended the accrual of 30 minutes of only moderate-intensity exercise performed on the majority of days of the week. Problematically, an adverse result of such guidelines is that some individuals and healthcare professionals believe that vigorous physical activity is not required for optimal health or the prevention and management of disease.

Since increasing benefits occur with concomitant increasing quantity and quality of physical activity, it is essential to consider the application of one or more of this vast number of physical activity modalities and their unique design elements to ensure optimal health promotion and disease prevention [11]. Establishing the most suitable combination of these elements is key to the success of an exercise programme in terms of health promotion, disease prevention and rehabilitation. Further, both the setting (i.e., school or workplace) and population (i.e., children or elderly community-dwelling adults) additionally complicates the determination of the elements [44].

Although, physical activity prescription has become an important public health issue, at an individual, practice or organisational level, there tends to be a focus on a single type of physical activity to improve health, and prevent or manage disease [37]. This is despite overwhelming evidence demonstrating that it is essential to undertake physical activity that promotes cardiorespiratory fitness, muscular fitness (including muscular strength and endurance), body composition, flexibility, and balance, not just one of these [37]. In general, the ACSM recommends that healthy adults perform aerobic training at 60–80% heart rate maximum, for 30–60 minutes a session, 3–5 days a week and resistance training be performed at 60–80% one-repetition maximum, using eight to 10 large muscle exercises, for eight to 12 repetitions and two to three sets, 2–3 days a week. According to the ACSM, to ensure optimal health and disease prevention, flexibility training should also be performed for 10–15 minutes twice a week and neuromotor training two to three times a week [45].

However, it is essential to note that this prescription may be considered overly simplified since programme design is additionally complicated by the level of fitness at the onset of the programme (i.e., beginner, intermediate or established). Further, when replicating and adapting physical activity programmes in a variety of public health settings, it is essential to consider the specific elements within an exercise programme design. When considering aerobic activities, modality (e.g., walking, running, swimming, cycling, and jumping), frequency, duration, and intensity need to be taken into consideration, while volume, intensity, tempo, rest intervals, and frequency need to be considered in resistance activities and whether muscle strength, muscle endurance, power and/or hypertrophy are the outcomes. The incorporation of flexibility activities into home, school and workplace physical activity programmes can lead to an enhanced overall health and well-being. However, the modality (e.g., static, or dynamic), stretch duration, and intensity all need to be considered. It is due to this sheer diversity of variables affecting physical activity public health programme interventions that an increased focus on training physical activity public health specialists or the development of guidelines and policies related to a formal referral scheme to qualified exercise specialists once established disease and multiple manifest risk factor for disease are present to appropriately manipulate the programme design elements to attain positive outcomes.

In this regard, although there is a need to build community- and population-wide capacity based on existing literature, there is a need to move away from a solely a behavioural science approach focusing on individuals, and rather to a systems approach that focuses on populations and the complex interactions among the correlates of physical inactivity [39, 40]. This is because the role of a variety of health professionals in prescribing appropriate physical activity or referrals to their clients, patients, children, and employees is vital to increasing global physical activity levels, which in turn, would enhance physical and mental health and well-being, and the prevention and management of key non-communicable diseases (NCDs).

The development, identification, and monitoring of approaches to promoting physical activity as a public health imperative in communities, schools, and workplaces, and at a population level need to be explored [46]. However, such approaches and recommendations need to be based on the principles of inclusive and engaged partnerships between various stakeholders such as members of community, investigators, healthcare professionals, and policy makers. More research is needed to identify factors influencing who receives physical activity interventions and how interventions are selected for communities and populations [47, 48]. Further, there is an increased need for all health professional, not just physiotherapists, Biokineticists, and exercise physiologists to (1) understand specific activities and interventions that they can incorporate as part of routine care that can prevent physical inactivity, (2) think about the resources and services available in their communities that can assist the community to become active, (3) how to measure their impact and value of their own contribution, and (4) understand and make use of physical activity referral schemes to suitably qualified health care professionals.

7. Conclusions

Physical inactivity is a major global issue. The benefits of regular physical activity as a public health intervention require health professionals to become aware and competent in prescribing it to promote wellbeing and prevent ill health as part of their everyday practice. Due to the increasing global incidence of NCDs and its scientific efficacy, physical activity has increasingly been included into public health initiatives.

However, there remains significant deficiencies policies, practice, and engagement as evidenced by the ever-increasing prevalence of physical inactivity. Thus, it is recommended that more emphasis be placed on the importance of physical activity on both our physical and mental health from a young age into advanced age, while considering specific and vulnerable populations to ensure equality. Political will is required to encourage health professionals and government alike to include physical activity into the fabric of public health, including schools, communities, and workplaces. This is because the prescription of physical activity by a variety of health professionals is critical to improve health, and prevent and manage chronic disease considering their trusted relationships with patients, families, and communities. Future work is needed related to the scalability of community- and population-wide physical activity intervention programmes.

Acknowledgements

The authors would like to acknowledge the contributions made by the Non-Communicable Disease Intervention Research Unit (NCDIRU).

Conflict of interest

The authors declare no conflict of interest.

Author details

Ina Shaw[1], Musa L. Mathunjwa[2] and Brandon S. Shaw[1]*

1 School of Sport, Rehabilitation and Exercise Sciences, University of Essex, Colchester, Essex, UK

2 Department of Human Movement Science, University of Zululand, Kwadlangezwa, South Africa

*Address all correspondence to: b.shaw@essex.ac.uk

References

[1] World Health Organization (WHO). Global recommendations on physical activity for health. 2009. Available at: http://www.who.int/ncds/prevention/physical-activity/en/ [Accessed: March 13, 2023]

[2] Avila-Palencia I. The effects of transport mode use on self-perceived health, mental health, and social contact measures: A cross-sectional and longitudinal study. Environment International. 2018;**120**:199-206. DOI: 10.1016/j.envint.2018.08.002

[3] World Health Organisation (WHO). Physical activity. Available at: https://www.who.int/news-room/fact-sheets/detail/physical-activity [Accessed: March 27, 2023]

[4] Warburton DE, Bredin SS. Reflections on physical activity and health: What should we recommend? Canadian Journal of Cardiology. 2016;**32**:495-504. DOI: 10.1016/j.cjca.2016.01.024

[5] Warburton DE, Bredin SS, Jamnik V, et al. Consensus on Evidence-Based Preparticipation Screening and Risk Stratification. New York City, NY: Springer Publishing Company; 2016. pp. 53-102

[6] Booth FW, Roberts CK, Laye MJ. Lack of exercise is a major cause of chronic diseases. Comprehensive Physiology. 2012;**2**(2):1143-1211. DOI: 10.1002/cphy.c110025

[7] Franklin BA, Billecke S. Putting the benefits and risks of aerobic exercise in perspective. Current Sports Medicine Reports. 2012;**11**(4):201-208. DOI: 10.1249/JSR.0b013e31825dabd4

[8] Bredin SS, Jamnik V, Gledhill N, Warburton DE. Effective Pre-Participation Screening and Risk Stratification. Health-Related Exercise Prescription for the Qualified Exercise Professional. 6th ed. Vancouver: Health & Fitness Society of BC; 2016. pp. 1-30

[9] Wasfy MM, Baggish AL. Exercise dose in clinical practice. Circulation. 2016;**133**:2297-2313

[10] Warburton DER, Bredin SSD, Zibadi S, Watson RR. Lost in Translation: What Does the Physical Activity and Health Evidence Actually Tell us? Lifestyle in Heart Health and Disease. San Diego, CA: Elsevier; 2017

[11] Mendes R, Sousa N, Barata JL. Actividade física e saúde pública: recomendações para a prescrição de exercício. Acta Medica Portugal. 2011;**24**(6):1025-1030. DOI: 10.20344/amp.1412

[12] Shaw BS, Brown GA, Shaw I. Importance of resistance training in the management of cardiovascular disease risk. In: Chahine J, editor. Cardiovascular Risk Factors. London, UK, London, United Kingdom: IntechOpen Publishers; 2021

[13] Harris MA. The relationship between physical inactivity and mental wellbeing: Findings from a gamification-based community-wide physical activity intervention. Health Psychology Open. 2018;**5**(1):2055102917753853. DOI: 10.1177/2055102917753853

[14] Fourie M, Gildenhuys GM, Shaw I, Shaw BS, Toriola AL, Goon DT. Effects of a mat Pilates program on flexibility in elderly women. Medicina dello Sport. 2013;**66**(4):545-553. DOI: 10.7727/wimj.2012.107

[15] Goon DT, Toriola AL, Shaw BS, Amusa LO, Khoza LB, Shaw I. Body fat percentage of urban south African children: Implications for health and fitness. West Indian Medical Journal. 2013;**62**(7):545-553

[16] Shaw BS, Shaw I, Brown GA. Self-reported dietary intake following endurance, resistance and concurrent endurance and resistance training. Journal of Sports Science & Medicine. 2008;**7**(2):255-259

[17] Shaw I, Shaw BS, Brown GA. Concurrent training and pulmonary function in smokers. International Journal of Sports Medicine. 2011;**32**(10):776-780. DOI: 10.1055/s-0031-1277214

[18] Peluso MA, Guerra de Andrade LH. Physical activity and mental health: The association between exercise and mood. Clinics. 2005;**60**(1):61-70. DOI: 10.1590/s1807-59322005000100012

[19] Nuzum H, Stickel A, Corona M, Zeller M, Melrose RJ, Wilkins SS. Potential benefits of physical activity in MCI and dementia. Behavioral Neurology. 2020;**2020**(12):7807856. DOI: 10.1155/2020/7807856

[20] Erickson KI, Hillman C, Stillman CM, Ballard RM, Bloodgood B, Conroy DE, et al. Physical activity, cognition, and brain outcomes: A review of the 2018 physical activity guidelines. Medicine and Science in Sports and Exercise. 2019;**51**(6):1242-1251. DOI: 10.1249/MSS.0000000000001936

[21] Markotić V, Pokrajčić V, Babić M, Radančević D, Grle M, Miljko M, et al. The positive effects of running on mental health. Psychiatria Danubina. 2020;**32**(Suppl 2):233-235

[22] Kandola A, Ashdown-Franks G, Hendrikse J, Sabiston CM, Stubbs B. Physical activity and depression: Towards understanding the antidepressant mechanisms of physical activity. Neuroscience and Biobehavioral Reviews. 2019;**107**:525-539. DOI: 10.1016/j.neubiorev.2019.09.040

[23] Pearce M, Garcia L, Abbas A, Strain T, Schuch FB, Golubic R, et al. Association between physical activity and risk of depression: A systematic review and meta-analysis. JAMA Psychiatry. 2022;**79**(6):550-559. DOI: 10.1001/jamapsychiatry.2022.0609

[24] Paluska SA, Schwenk TL. Physical activity and mental health: Current concepts. Sports Medicine. 2000;**29**(3):167-180. DOI: 10.2165/00007256-200029030-00003

[25] Viru A, Smirnova T. Health promotion and exercise training. Sports Medicine. 1995;**19**(2):123-136. DOI: 10.2165/00007256-199519020-00004

[26] Nystoriak MA, Bhatnagar A. Cardiovascular effects and benefits of exercise. Frontiers in Cardiovascular Medicine. 2018;**28**(5):135. DOI: 10.3389/fcvm.2018.00135

[27] Shaw BS, Lloyd R, Da Silva M, Coetzee D, Moran J, Waterworth SPW, et al. German volume training for health promotion: Acute vasopressor, pulmonary and metabolic responses. Frontiers in Physiology. 2022;**13**:1025017. DOI: 10.3389/fphys.2022.102501

[28] Shaw BS, Turner S, Shaw I. Comparison of muscle endurance and hypertrophy resistance training on cardiovascular disease risk in smokers. Asian Journal of Sports Medicine. 2021;**12**(1):1-6. DOI: 10.5812/asjsm.106589

[29] Taylor CB, Sallis JF, Needle R. The relation of physical activity and exercise to mental health. Public Health Reports. 1985;**100**(2):195-202

[30] Mikkelsen K, Stojanovska L, Polenakovic M, Bosevski M, Apostolopoulos V. Exercise and mental health. Maturitas. 2017;**106**:48-56. DOI: 10.1016/j.maturitas.2017.09.003

[31] Tzu-Wei L, Yu-Min K. Exercise benefits brain function: The monoamine connection. Brain Science. 2013;**3**(1):39-53. DOI: 10.3390/brainsci3010039

[32] Spiteri K, Broom D, Bekhet AH, de Caro JX, Laventure B, Grafton K. Barriers and motivators of physical activity participation in middle-aged and older-adults - a systematic review. Journal of Aging and Physical Activity. 2019;**27**(4):929-944. DOI: 10.1123/japa.2018-0343

[33] Hou Y, Zhai C, Chen X, Li W. The effect of the street environment on two types of essential physical activity in industrial neighborhoods from the perspective of public health: A study from the Harbin low-income population health survey, China. BMC Public Health. 2022;**22**(1):2201. DOI: 10.1186/s12889-022-14533-7

[34] Lawrence KE, Shaw I, Shaw BS. Hemodynamic changes in normotensive overweight and obese individuals following home-based calisthenics training. African Journal for Physical, Health Education, Recreation and Dance. 2014;**2014**(2):82-90

[35] Heath GW, Levine D. Physical activity and public health among people with disabilities: Research gaps and recommendations. International Journal of Environmental Research and Public Health. 2022;**19**(16):10436. DOI: 10.3390/ijerph191610436

[36] Shaw BS, Shaw I. Resistance training as a countermeasure for key non-communicable diseases in low-resource settings: A review. Asian. Journal of Sports Medicine. 2021;**12**(1):1-8. DOI: 10.5812/asjsm.106588

[37] King AC. Community and public health approaches to the promotion of physical activity. Medicine and Science in Sports and Exercise. 1994;**26**(11):1405-1412. DOI: 10.1249/00005768-199411000-00017

[38] Goon DT, Toriola AL, Shaw BS. Screening for body weight disorders in Nigerian children using contrasting definitions. Obesity Reviews. 2009;**11**(7):508-515. DOI: 10.1111/j.1467-789X.2009.00682.x

[39] Shandu NM, Mathunjwa ML, Shaw BS, Shaw I. Effects of high-intensity interval training and continuous aerobic training on health-fitness, health related quality of life, and psychological measures in college-aged smokers. International Journal of Environmental Research and Public Health. 2022;**20**(1):653. DOI: 10.3390/ijerph20010653

[40] Kohl HW, Craig CL, Lambert EV, Inoue S, Alkandari JR, Leetongin G, et al. The pandemic of physical inactivity: global action for public health. Lancet. 2012;**380**(9838):294-305. DOI: 10.1016/S0140-6736(12)60898-8

[41] Physical Activity in the Workplace. Available from: https://evidence.nihr.ac.uk/themedreview/moving-matters-interventions-to-increase-physical-activity/ [Accessed: May 10, 2023]

[42] Morar D, Coopoo Y, Shaw I, Shaw BS. Health and fitness attitudes and lifestyle habits of urban children in South Africa. African Journal for Physical Health

Education, Recreation and Dance. 2014;**20**:102-112

[43] Sumaira H, Malik HB, Suggs LS. A systematic review of workplace health promotion interventions for increasing physical activity. British Journal of Health Psychology. 2014;**19**(1):149-180. DOI: 10.1111/bjhp.12052

[44] Warburton DE, Charlesworth S, Ivey A, et al. A systematic review of the evidence for Canada's physical activity guidelines for adults. International Journal of Behavioural Nutrition and Physical Activity. 2010;**7**:39

[45] Cooney JK, Law R, Matschke V, Lemmey AB. Benefits of exercise in rheumatoid arthritis. Journal of Aging Research. 2011;**10**:681-640. DOI: 10.4061/2011/681640

[46] Goon DT, Toriola AL, Shaw BS. Sex differences in body fatness in Nigerian children. African Journal for Physical, Health Education, Recreation and Dance. 2007;**13**(3):294-305. DOI: 10.4314/ajpherd.v13i3.24773

[47] Goon DT, Toriola AL, Shaw BS, Amusa LO. Centripetal fat patterning in South African children. Pakistan Journal of Medical Sciences. 2011;**27**(4):832-836. DOI: 10.4314/ajpherd.v15i4.49553

[48] Semin K, Stahlnecker AC IV, Heelan K, Brown GA, Shaw BS, Shaw I. Discrepancy between training, competition and laboratory measures of maximum heart rate in NCAA division 2 distance runners. Journal of Sports Science & Medicine. 2008;**7**(4):455-460

Chapter 2

Modern Healthy Lifestyle Program or the Opportunity to Develop Modern Health Consciousness

Annamária Juhász and Péter Habil Fritz

Abstract

Our modern world presents us with ever new challenges that lead to new solutions in all aspects of our lives. Innovation is also evident in our social arrangements, which, similar to the introduction of a new product to the market, entails strong marketing activities in order to be success. Social innovation combined with a social marketing school can bring about very effective social change. This study presents a social innovation that can serve as a pilot project in the field of health promotion. This pilot project is built on the model of holistic health consciousness and responsibility which is a special health promotion and primary prevention example. Within the program, health promotion centers will be established in four locations (Budapest, Miskolc, Szikszó, and Szeged), where natural ingredients and modern technological tools will provide personalized services for primary and secondary prevention and population health promotion.

Keywords: modern age, holistic, health consciousness, responsibility, primary prevention, health promotion, social innovation, social marketing

1. Introduction

Modern age health consciousness is in focus because our modern world has never had such a range of technological tools at its disposal, and we have never had to deal with such a level of stress as we do today. The WHO definition of health has been expanded by the COVID-19 epidemic, and also the growing power of new health-related knowledge and the abundance of health industry products and services have created a kind of chaos in the maintenance of health. The fundamental question arises as to whether the individual is solely responsible for his or her own health or whether society's responsibility should also be interpreted in a broader sense. Both the health consciousness models and the empirical survey show the role of the environment and the influencing actors. (Actors of the social spheres, which can be individuals as well as organizations.)

However, neither individuals nor environmental actors were sufficiently aware of the extent of their responsibility. In a holistic approach, taking responsibility for health can be interpreted and extended to the environmental actors surrounding the individual. A paradigm shift is needed both at the level of the individual and at the level of societal actors. In 2016, the model of holistic health consciousness and responsibility was created and is now presented in a streamlined form precisely because it reflects the holistic approach along multiple that forms the basis for the development of modern health consciousness.

1.1 The model for holistic health consciousness and responsibility

The holistic health consciousness and responsibility model reflects a multiactor and specific stakeholder management approach. It starts from the problem that individuals' health consciousness and responsibility must be strengthened in order to increase overall societal well-being. The model identifies the stakeholders who can support and develop individuals' health consciousness without harming their own interests.

The holistic health consciousness and responsibility model are holistic in several ways (**Figure 1**). First of all, it assumes the harmony of body-mind-spirit at the level of the individual. We interpret the state of health as the continuous balance of this threefold unity, that is, as a sequence of momentary states. Second, the model is holistic in that it includes the social actors who are able to influence and even intervene in individual health, thus becoming a social actor. Third, it is holistic because it integrates the concept of health into sustainable development, that is, it considers health as one of the starting points and, on the other hand, as one of the outcomes of sustainable development [1].

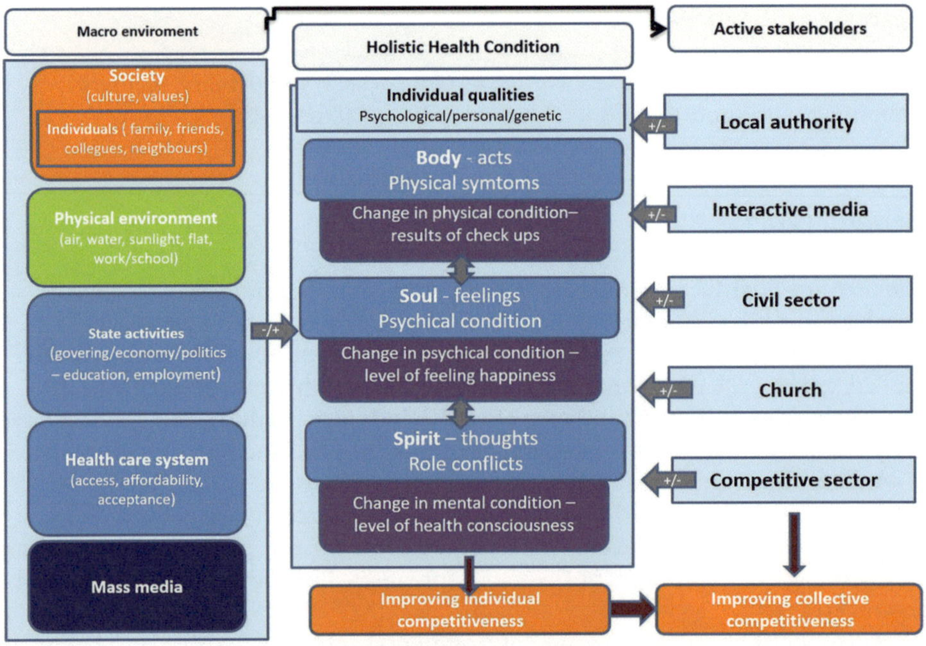

Figure 1.
The model of holistic health consciousness and responsibility 2022. Source: Mató-Juhász et al. [2].

1.2 Individual responsibility

An essential element of holistic health is individual responsibility. Individual responsibility encompasses lifestyle and various health maintenance factors that can affect physical, mental, and spiritual state, as well as social relationships. To all of this is added the responsibility of the individual in various roles:

- As a private person, the individual can influence the health of others, for example, as a partner, parent, friend, or member of the local community.
- As an employee, health-conscious behavior is also important, that is, which means, on the one hand, compliance with health and safety regulations, employer expectations of a healthy work environment and health-protective work tasks, and on the other hand, ensuring that the individual's engagement in work does not lead to damage to health (e.g., workaholism, burnout).
- In addition, the individual also plays an important role as a consumer, so that health-conscious behavior also means a kind of responsible consumption, which should also be extended to environmentally conscious and media-conscious consumption [1].

1.3 The macro environment of health

In creating the model, we assumed that a number of macro-environmental factors have a promoting or inhibiting effect on the health of individuals. We defined five main factors:

- One of the most important factors is society (the person of family and friends is particularly important), which represents the values and culture of the particular environment.
- The next important factor that has a great impact on the health of the individuals is the physical environment itself: air quality, drinking water quality and access, and solar radiation, Schumann resonance, housing conditions, school, and working conditions.
- Government and its activities are another critical factor in the health of individuals. This group includes the areas of politics and administration, as these largely determine the options available to the individual.
- The health care system is closely related to government activities but is mentioned as a separate category because of its impact on health, especially physical health.
- Nowadays, the media are extremely important among the influencing factors [1].

1.4 Stakeholders/actors

The model also includes the stakeholders that have an impact on the health of individuals as intervention actors, that is, deliberate actions that support the health of individuals can be associated with stakeholders as actors:

- In terms of health, the community is a stakeholder that can become an intervention actor with regulations to protect and promote health.
- The media, including social media, can intervene as actors by raising health consciousness. This can include drawing attention to health-promoting options and shaping opinion for more positive acceptance of it.
- The civil sector and the church can become intervention actors through their various opinion shaping and support activities.
- The corporate sector can become a very significant intervention actor, especially based on its corporate social responsibility, if it offers healthy products and services to its customers, provides a cafeteria system for its employees, organizes and mediates cultural programs, provides health-promoting working conditions, strengthens the feeling of appreciation, and provides health-promoting and regenerating opportunities [1].

Therefore, if we examine the individual's self-responsibility in terms of maintaining and restoring his or her holistic state of health, we can conclude that he or she must have a wide range of knowledge about himself or herself and the influence of the environment and others. In the service of health, self-knowledge gains its true weight and importance when the individual (1) has sufficient knowledge of the functioning of his body and continuously monitors it by means of various (screening) tests, (2) understands and relates his mental state and physical reactions and is able to recognize and process his or her feelings, (3) is able to define and understand his or her various roles in relation to others and is able to define and maintain the boundaries of his or her various roles in a way that does not harm the health of others [1].

2. Methodology and results

During the review of the topic, it became clear that the increase in health consciousness will be examined according to the model presented above.

Thus, I did a qualitative research, document, and content analysis, examining the occurrence of the term "improving health consciousness" in Hungarian professional materials. It can be stated that increasing health consciousness means complex health improvement, using modern technologies.

2.1 Health improvement in the modern age

So the modern health-conscious person sees and lives in this complex system, so he expects positive responsibility for himself, his environment, and others. Thus, the responsibility of the macro-environment and stakeholders is to consciously create a supportive environment for the individual. The health-promoting environment represents a novel approach to health promotion.

Health promotion refers to all nontherapeutic interventions that promote the maintenance, development, and improvement of health and the resolution of health problems of a behavioral and/or environmental nature. Therefore, health promotion integrates the existing substrategies of health information, health education and teaching, self-help, and prevention into a single concept. It also emphasizes the need for interdisciplinarity and crossing sectoral boundaries, the consideration of living and working conditions, and opportunities for public participation [3].

In terms of health, development means "improving" health, that is, providing information, support, and the prioritizing health issues at both the individual and society levels [3, 4]. The basic goal of health promotion is to enable people to gain more control over the factors that affect their lives and health.

Health is a positive concept that encompasses both individual and social resources beyond "physical fitness" [3]. The central element of the definition is the issue of control, which expresses the active nature of health promotion. The so-called "prevention" of diseases of civilization is not possible without the proper motivation and active participation of the individual and community.

The so-called "epidemiological" epochal change – the shift in the spectrum of leading causes of death from infectious diseases to chronic, noninfectious diseases – also required a paradigm shift in medicine and medical practice.

The World Health Organization's (WHO) definition of health promotion World Health Organization (WHO) Definition Of Health - Public Health aptly states, "Health promotion is the process of enabling people to exercise increasing influence (control) over the factors that determine their health and to improve their own health status."

The outlined perspective follows from the concept of health and also includes the extent to which an individual or group is able to realize their desires and satisfy their needs; on the other hand, they can change their environment and cope with the task of environmental protection. Health is therefore seen as a resource in daily life, not as a goal in life. This positive sounding formulation emphasizes social and personal resources as well as physical capacity/endurance, that is, fitness of the individual [3, 5].

The fundamental aspect and goal of health promotion is to empower and enable people to pay more attention to the factors that affect their lives and health, in Hungarian: "to take more care of their health" [3, 5].

The new approach to health promotion must bring a renewal, where health promotion increasingly becomes a kind of lifestyle program that extends to the whole; it includes old and young, men and women, healthy and sick. The most important element of health promotion with a new approach is personal development, which enables you to find joy in life and improve the quality of life. In this change of attitude, the results of multidisciplinary health-related research and their effective application must play a key role [3].

2.2 Examples in health improvement in the modern age

In Hungary, best practices consist of connecting professional areas, where health improvement is managed in holistic, complex way. This means that individual health plans, based on lifestyle medicine, are made by examining the areas of nutrition, exercise, and mental hygiene. The environmental effects are examined, and the environmental actors are also considered actors who can be addressed. At the same time, in implementation, health education typically focuses on the individual responsibility. There are already examples where the environmental actors cooperate in order to improve health.

An example is the oncology prehabilitation program in the Hungarian health care system, which works from the diagnosis of cancer to the active oncological treatment. This program professionally prepares the patient and his environment for the treatments, and the modifiable risk factors within the scope of supply [6]. In this protocol as well, the professionally holistic approach is applied (simultaneous analysis and modification of nutrition, physical therapy, mental hygiene areas), and actors who provide active intervention in some area, such as pastors, civil society, social workers, are already appearing [7].

Another example is a workplace health improvement, which shows that the holistic approach is used by the Hungarian Police. They connect the field of medicine, psychology, and law enforcement for the most effective health improvement. The purpose of the Life-Strength-Health Program is to maintain health support programs operating at the police, to standardize its implementation principles at the national level, and to introduce new programs [8].

The eight pillars of workplace recreation and health improvement at the Hungarian Police:

1. Healthy eating at workplaces.

2. Organizing health days.

3. Once a month, holding interactive educational lectures for the staff with the participation of healthcare professionals.

4. Individualized health counseling during fitness tests.

5. Possible participation in civil screening tests.

6. Providing discounted sports opportunities for the staff.

7. Broadcasting of computer presentations and health improvement videos on TV sets in the waiting rooms of health services.

8. Conducting psychological trainings for personnel.

As we can see there is no such complex increasing health consciousness example in Hungary that can be used for social innovation framework. This study shows a program which is built on the model of holistic health consciousness and responsibility.

3. Modern healthy lifestyle program as a method to increase modern health consciousness

This rather complex model also shows that the basis of health consciousness is the responsible use of information and its functional integration into the daily routine. Putting the holistic model of health consciousness and responsibility into practice is the Modern Healthy Lifestyle Program, which is both social innovation and social marketing.

We see the improvement of people's health effectively implemented by creating a business community whose activities are to produce and provide products and services that support people's holistic health in a scientifically and professionally proven way, and we carry out their marketing communications. To this end, we see the implementation of the program in collaboration with companies that have many years of experience in the field of health, working with professional associations and civil organizations that are authoritative in scientific and professional guidelines and certifications. In addition to all this, all actors are capable of interdisciplinarity, that is, of working in partnership with other areas of science and other sectors under the auspices of social innovation.

The research and development pillar of the Modern Healthy Lifestyle Program cooperates with renowned representatives of many scientific fields and industries, for example, medicine, nutrition, sports science, health industry, environmental protection, energy industry, food industry, beauty industry. Each of these areas in itself is a key factor for the successful implementation of the program, but in its complexity leads to synergies. The education and implementation pillar of the program brings the results of the previous R&D pillar into people's everyday lives through various products and services. The communication pillar of the program draws attention to the results of the previous two pillars.

3.1 The main elements of the program

1. Providing project preparation and project management

2. Creating the Modern Healthy Lifestyle Innovation Research Center (MHL Innovation Research Center), expanding human resources for research, and creating administrative infrastructure conditions:

    - Creating of a Health Care Development Innovation Fund to finance research, studies, and start-ups

3. Modern Healthy Lifestyle Product Development Center (MHL Development Center) R&D-based product development of healthy foods and dietary supplements, development of production technologies, creation of infrastructural conditions, accreditation.

4. Establishment of Modern Healthy Lifestyle Selfness Centers

    - Establishment of preventive – holistic health centers in the cities of Miskolc, Szeged, Budapest – application of franchise business policy based on the synergy of bioresonance, natural healing factors and modern technology, and operation of lifestyle clubs.

    - Development of a diagnostic measuring station for an example project of health tourism in Szikszó.

5. Establishment of the Modern Healthy Lifestyle Social Innovation Center (MHL Social Innovation Center), expansion of human resources in the areas of teaching and media, and creation of administrative infrastructural conditions.

    - Marketing, communication (podcast series on recreation and health promotion in cooperation with the Central and Eastern European Recreation Society)

    - Education, trainings: presenting of development results, monitoring social needs, providing social experiences, strengthening belonging, providing access to lectures and presentations online.

    - Conference presentations and scientific publications

- Dissemination
- Organization of events

3.2 Implementer of the program

Another guarantee of successful implementation is a team that manages and owns companies operating on stable foundations with, several years or decades of professional experience and a good reputation at national and international level. Cooperation partners include higher education institutions and civil organizations (**Figure 2**).

3.3 Strategic partners

3.3.1 Responsible for the research Center for Health Economics and Innovation Fund

Med-Econ Human Szolgáltató Kft was established in July 2006 as a health and economic consulting company. Its main field of activity is the planning, preparation and management of planned and ongoing developments, investments and professional programs in the field of health care, health technology assessment (HTA), strategy and project management, preparation of business plans, development of service profiles for primary and speciality health care, and the development of related professional concepts. Through the analysis and research of domestic and foreign healthcare and health insurance systems, the company considers the development and promotion of healthcare system as its mission. The company also has an international presence (med-econ.hu).

3.3.2 Responsible for the recreation points area

When the SuperFoods team was established in 2013, they aimed to improve people's health and lifestyle. They strive to ensure that clients who come to them can access as many services as possible in one place, which helps improve their health. Initially, they worked

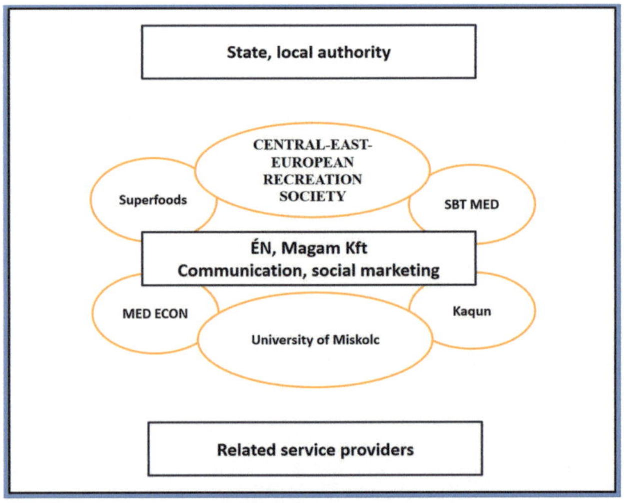

Figure 2.
The implementers of the modern healthy lifestyle program. Source: Own editing.

primarily with elite athletes, as for them nutrition plays a key role in preparing for competitions, building muscles properly and recovering. But their help is increasingly being sought by civilians whose goal is to lose weight, increase their fitness, or improve their overall quality of life. Their goal is to provide complex services with the help of competent professionals. Their focus is on health. They strive to improve the days of their clients, whether in top sports, at work, or in the way they feel about life (Superfoodteam.hu).

3.3.3 Kaqun water

The world's first oxygenated water was confirmed by clinical tests. Our story began in 2002 in Hungary. Its founder, Dr. Robert Lyons PhD. O.MD, set the goal of creating a product that could store and transport oxygen in a previously unknown way. With this idea, the special water was created that is now known worldwide as KAQUN. Unlike traditional oxygen therapies, KAQUN is unique in that it uses a method of oxygen delivery that focuses on our body's ability to balance low oxygen pressure in the tissues with the high oxygen content of KAQUN water. KAQUN water is not average purified drinking water, as the oxygen it contains is intended to support any condition that benefits from an increased supply of oxygen to the tissues. Regular consumption of KAQUN water improves quality of life and helps the immune system function, detoxifies, refreshes, and energizes. In addition, it helps with physical and mental performance and regeneration.

3.3.3.1 It may support our immune system

Oxygen is a crucial element for our cells and our body. Without it, our body and cells will become less efficient to maintain optimal physical and mental condition. With KAQUN water, we may support our cells with sufficient oxygen to improve our overall well-being.

3.3.3.2 It may decrease hypoxia

Hypoxia, also known as oxygen deficiency, is a medical term used to describe a condition in which our cells do not receive enough oxygen. Here, it is key to differentiate between the oxygen supply to the blood and the cell, as even in the case of a perfect blood oxygen supply, oxygen deficiency in the cells can occur. By consuming KAQUN water, we can enhance both our cellular and blood oxygen level.

3.3.3.3 It may improve performance

Several articles have investigated the importance of oxygen supply on athletes' performance, and the results all pretty much conclude that lacking oxygen not only affects sports performance but also physiological function too.

By drinking KAQUN water we could enhance performance under intense exercise since, during activity, the main fuel of our body (glycogen) is delivered to the cells by oxygen. Therefore, by improving the oxygen supply, we can improve our fuel delivery mechanism for better perforce.

3.3.3.4 It may improve recovery

Better performance does not just depend on the amount of work done. If our oxygen supply is inadequate, our cells will use 16 times more energy to regenerate.

This process increases the production of lactic acid in the muscles, resulting in muscle pain and fatigue. By consuming KAQUN water, we can reduce lactic acid production for more effective regeneration.

3.3.3.5 Improve memory and mood

Research has shown that even a mild lack of oxygen can impair memory and well-being from children to the elderly. Our brain uses most of the oxygen we breathe to maintain basic functions for our survival, therefore, improving our oxygen supply can enhance all brain function (KAQUN.hu).

3.3.4 Responsible for the range of medical health points

SBT MED is a self-care system with an international medical background that incorporates cutting-edge twenty-first century technology. The quantum technology of the ZYTO™ scanning manual cradle serves as the foundation for conscious self-care that complements traditional health care. The essence of ZYTO™ technology is biocommunication scanning. By measuring the body's galvanic skin response, the ZYTO™ health assessment provides us with "molecular depth," personalized map of our body's condition. It provides a report on the root of the problems that have occurred. ZYTO™ manual cradle technology is based on sound scientific principles: Patented software (US Food and Drug Administration (FDA) approved devices). (sbtmed.com).

3.3.5 Responsible for social innovation and social marketing

ÉN, Magam Kft was founded in 2011 to raise awareness of holistic health. PR and Communication implement their main activities with social marketing tools. The company targets individuals, companies, and institutions. The main profile of the company: development and implementation of PR and marketing strategies, production of media content, media management, communication and self-development trainings, consultations on work–life balance and well-being at work (enmagamkft.hu).

3.4 Organization responsible for the professional framework of prevention

3.4.1 The central-east-European recreation society (Abbrievated: Garden) is the XXI

It was founded in 2010 as a social challenge of the twentieth century.

The society, which also extends to neighboring countries, is aimed at professionals who research, teach, and work in the recreational and frontier field, students studying the profession, and anyone interested in healthy living and health promotion.

The aim of the NGO is to conduct scientific research that addresses the frontier areas of leisure (sports science, health science, nutrition science, sports psychology, education science, and economics – tourism). It integrates the latest professional knowledge into its educational and consulting services. Active participation in scientific conferences, elaboration and publication of professional materials focused on leisure-related health promotion, prevention of diseases education, and training. Organization and conduct free recreation-based health promotion programs that help individuals, families, and communities to improve their quality of life by regularly engaging in active recreation. Emphasizing the characteristic "recreation is ageless and boundless," which is used to emphasize collaboration, acceptance, and shared experiences between generations and nations.

Collaborating with the nonprofit and for-profit sectors, providing professional coordination as an umbrella organization to support quality services inside and outside the workplace.

3.4.2 Recreation scientific magazine

Reports quarterly on a high professional level about research results, trends, applied procedures, services, gastronomy, sports nutrition, and tourist attractions in the leisure sector and its peripheral areas (in Hungarian with English summary; and in English with a Hungarian summary) (recreationcentral.eu).

3.5 Organizations responsible for education

The University of Miskolc and the University of Szeged are the institutions where the strategic partners also act as senior lecturers, helping to shape and influence vocational training.

4. Discussion of results

The 2022 streamlined version of the Holistic Health Consciousness and Responsibility model represents the complex system that provides the theoretical framework for effective health promotion. The Modern Healthy Lifestyle Program can provide an answer to increasing health consciousness in the modern age. It is a social innovation model that formulates and implements a developmental concept based on its own research findings, builds on this with educational implementation, and finally focuses on integrated communication for audiences.

The MHL Program is an activity that can be understood as affiliate marketing (www.modernhealthylifestyle.hu).

Affiliate marketing is an area of online marketing that is less known in Hungary. The point is that content producers mediate conversions for advertisers and receive a predetermined commission from the price of the purchase. A real win-win situation for both parties: the advertiser increases his revenue, and the content producer effectively sells his surfaces.

At the same time, it also means a network of prevention-focused health centers based on stress management, suitable for personal consultation.

By promoting healthy lifestyles and improving quality of life, preventive health centers help to address and counteract stress caused by individual lifestyles, while validating the results of health economics and health technology research/development on a global scale.

Using a holistic approach (physical–spiritual–mental–social), the parts of the program increase the number of healthy years of life and lead to a positive experience for the Hungarian and foreign clients who use and apply the project results, using the tools of the modern age. Taking into account the preventive focus and building on the personal responsibility of the individual, it appears as a novelty that by putting the human being and his environment (living space, workplace) in the center, innovative technologies of the health industry, air, sunlight, water, nutrition play a crucial role something about the effect of Schumann Resonance on health.

Author details

Annamária Juhász[1*] and Péter Habil Fritz[2]

1 Faculty of Economics, Institute of Marketing and Tourism, University of Miskolc, Miskolc, Hungary

2 Faculty of Health Sciences, Institute of Applied Health Sciences, University of Miskolc, Miskolc, Hungary

*Address all correspondence to: annamaria.juhasz@uni-miskolc.hu

References

[1] Juhász A. A modern kori egészségtudatosság, avagy mit is értünk ma holisztikán?= modern health consciousness, or what do we mean by holistic today? Recreation. 2022;**12**(3):30-33. DOI: 10.21486/recreation.2022.12.3.5

[2] Mató-Juhász A, Kiss-Tóth E, Szegedi K. Holistic health model of sustainable development. European Scientific Journal. 2016;**12**(21):227-239, 13 p

[3] Péter F, Ernő J, Péter D. Mészáros Judit: A munkahelyi egészségfejlesztés európai gyakorlata. Budapesti Népegészségügy, XXXV. évf. 4.szám. 2004:324-330

[4] Ewles L, Simnett I. Promoting Health – A Practical Guide. 1999. Medicina KönyvkKiadó. 1999. ISBN: 9632425545

[5] Ewles L, Simnett I. Promoting Health – A Practical Guide. 2013. Medicina Könyvkiadó. 1999. ISBN: 9789632264332

[6] Santa Mina D, Van Rooijen SJ, Minnella EM, et al. Multiphasic prehabilitation across the cancer continuum: A narrative review and conceptual framework. Frontiers in Oncology. 2021;**10**:598425

[7] Furka A. Oncological prehabilitation. Orvosi Hetilap. 2022;**163**(50):1975-1981. DOI: 10.1556/650.2022.32646

[8] Tánczos Z, Sipos E, Szeles E, Witzing Z, Polácska E, Bognár J. Munkahelyi egészségfejlesztés a rendőrség személyi állományának körében. Belügyi Szemle. 2021;(2021/3. különszám):32-47. DOI: 10.38146/BSZ.SPEC.2021.3.2

Chapter 3

Participation as a Core Principle of Community Health Promotion: General Account and Examples

Alf Trojan, Christian Lorentz and Stefan Nickel

Abstract

One of the key principles of the Ottawa Charta is participation. Community health interventions should involve the community, i.e., residents and local actors. In Hamburg, we tried to put this principle into practice during a project initiated by the municipal health service in a disadvantaged quarter with about 3000 inhabitants. The contribution starts with an account of the meaning of participation in health promotion (1) and gives an overview of participation methods in general (2). The next part contains a short account of our project (3). Five examples are presented in part four: a survey with key actors and two approaches to listening to residents' perceptions of capacity building in the neighborhood. Another survey of residents was meant to explore the use of health promotion offers and the preparedness to get involved. The last example is the round table of local actors as a sort of steering committee for health promotion interventions (4). Key findings of the examples are: Surveys do result in valuable information for the local actors. The expressed willingness to participate is larger than the actual participation. Opportunities to participate (in surveys and at the round table) are welcome by local actors. In the last section we discuss the advantages, problems and some illusions concerning participation in health promotion (5).

Keywords: participation, resident survey, round table, disadvantaged area, Ottawa Charter

1. Introduction

In as early as 1986, the WHO's Ottawa Charter stressed the central importance of participation and civic involvement in the implementation of health promotion programs, policies, and activities. The normative demand for democratic involvement and the strengthening of civic communities, neighborhoods, and groups, but also of the individual citizen in terms of the development of personal competences and skills, pervades the entire text of the Ottawa Charter but is particularly emphasized in individual passages:

"Strengthen community action.

Health promotion works through concrete and effective community action in setting priorities, making decisions, planning strategies and implementing them to achieve better health. At the heart of this process is the empowerment of communities, their ownership and control of their own endeavors and destinies. Community development draws on existing human and material resources in the community to enhance self-help and social support, and to develop flexible systems for strengthening public participation and direction of health matters. This requires full and continuous access to information, learning opportunities for health, as well as funding support" [1].

Of course, this applies not only to the activation and participation of the envisaged target groups [2] in the population, but also to the leading actors in health policy programs and activities. Participation, sharing, civic involvement, cooperation, community action – whatever terminology is used or argued within this context – it tends to move away from the "top-down" approach and toward a more "bottom-up" approach. The advantages of bottom-up approaches are based on opportunities to participate and strong efforts to empower local communities. They have been demonstrated in a number of well-researched examples [3].

2. Methods and participatory instruments for community-based health promotion

The possibilities and methods for implementing this democratic right are as diverse as the levels of intensity of participation and civic involvement, if one wants to gradually approach the normative requirements as formulated by the WHO in its Ottawa Charter. In recent decades, different models, strategies, and procedures have been discussed, developed, and tested in practice in many policy areas and evaluated in subsequent scientific projects [4–6]. There is a wealth of experience from several decades of practical civic involvement and participation [3, 7], which has now also been extended to include the aspect of participation in health research [8–10]. A separate classification scheme is presented here as an example of the various similar models.

The ladder models for civic involvement in decision-making processes or participation in health promotion are helpful constructs for the discussion and evaluation processes involved in strategic planning of political programs and activities, which can also be transferred to programs for prevention and health promotion. The models try to make clear that real participation and involvement entail different levels of intensity with respect to authority to exert power. According to these models, it is therefore always necessary to determine how much decision-making power actually lies with the population groups involved and their legal actors in order to speak of participation, preliminary stages of participation, or nonparticipation. Participation is not understood as an either/or option but as a development process.

In addition to this normative and politically oriented assessment of participation and civic involvement, a number of practical and creative methods and procedures for the participation of citizens and/or professional actors have developed in recent decades within the framework of urban planning and redevelopment processes, from project development and action planning to the formulation and implementation of political programs in different fields of action and policy areas. In addition, significant momentum for the development and further development of procedures and methods also came from the field of health promotion and prevention, not least through the Gesunde Städte (Healthy Cities) project. The German Healthy Cities network has a so-called 9-Points-Program of self-commitments. This document has to

Traditional methods and instruments	Creative methods and instruments
• Oral or written surveying of a quantitative or qualitative nature	• Planning cell
• Bodies, advisory councils, committees	• Open space events
• Round tables	• Future workshop
• Networking institutions related to the particular fields of work	• Focus groups
• District conferences	• Research into the lived environment
• Town hall meetings	• Citizens' exhibition
• Consultations	• Planning for real
• Working groups	• Suggestion box
• Initiatives and pressure groups	• Neighborhood detectives
• And more	• Citizen tours/inspections
	• And more

Table 1.
Traditional and creative methods of communication and involvement.

be signed before becoming a member city. Point 5 requires that the city has to provide a framework that guarantees that all citizens "can participate in the shaping of healthy living conditions and environments." Point 7 requires, that in the steering committees of the cities there has to be at least one representative of local citizen initiatives or self-help groups.[1]

The list in **Table 1** provides a brief overview, without evaluation initially, of what can be "done today" in the areas of civic involvement and participation in the interests of the above-mentioned ladder models. The extent to which political decision-making processes can be influenced or even shaped shall not play a role at this point. It is important to note that participation and involvement always also require that the citizenry, or the particular neighborhoods or groups of the community concerned, generally have to be activated in some form in order to "participate" in participatory processes. This means that the methods and procedures used are always also about activation for participation and about the participatory process itself.

According to a study by the German Youth Institute [11] on the activation and participation of families, these methods and procedures can be differentiated between in terms of traditional and creative instruments of communication and involvement. These are listed in **Table 1** and supplemented for this paper by a number of other known participatory instruments.

In the socio-political process, for example, at the municipal level, a mix of traditional and creative instruments is often found, depending on the needs, the subject matter, and the desired solution to the upcoming problems and decisions.

The individual techniques, procedures, and methods mentioned here cannot and should not be discussed at this point. The focus of our remarks is intended, rather, to be on examples of participatory community-based health promotion as addressed and implemented in a disadvantaged district of Hamburg-Eimsbüttel by the local health office.

The practical project, which is accompanied by continuous research, was entitled "Lenzgesund" ("Lenzhealthy," tying in with the name of the district, "Lenzsiedlung" (the Lenz estate)).

[1] https://gesunde-staedte-netzwerk.de/wp-content/uploads/9-Punkte_Programm.pdf

3. General presentation of the practical project "Lenzgesund"

Almost in parallel to the district's inclusion in the Senate "Social District Development" program, the Hamburg-Eimsbüttel Health Office also began to contribute to the district's management in 2001 with its first health-promoting activities. These activities initially focused on the situation of young families and migrants, as the Lenzsiedlung is a large housing estate close to the city center that is home to very many children, mostly of foreign background.

Two years later, in the autumn of 2003, at the initiative of the health office, the first "Lenzgesund" round table was launched, which was intended, on the one hand, to contribute to networking among the actors and, on the other hand, to serve as an interface between the actors and the population. At the round table, three to four times a year, various institutions, and individuals from the health, education, and social sectors met in and around the Lenzsiedlung, with the aim of establishing health promotion and prevention as a priority field of action for district development.

A systematic prevention program entitled "Lenzgesund" was introduced by the health office in 2005, and has since been implemented and further developed together with other collaborative partners. The core of the dynamic concept of action is the organization and coordination of networked assistance around pregnancy, childbirth, and the first years of life, with the aim of improving health status with the active participation of the residents in the neighborhood. The idea is to make a small-scale contribution to equal social and health opportunities. The objectives in detail are:

- to improve the health situation in the neighborhood, especially for children and their parents;
- to develop a good health care structure in the vicinity of the settlement for the residents;
- to build and secure bridging structures between the available medical and social services and the health needs of the population;
- to promote networking activities within the framework of individual fields of action of the program; and
- to achieve collaboration between health and social care institutions and health promotion.

After several discussions at the round table (see below), the prevention program, which initially consisted of nine fields of action, was divided into seven fields of action (with individual subgoals and target groups) as well as two cross-cutting tasks that are to be integrated into all fields of action. These fields of action and cross-cutting tasks of the prevention program are:

1. Preparation for birth
2. Pregnancy/parenthood among minors (services for teenagers)
3. Support after birth and during the first year of life

4. Vaccination

5. Early assistance, early intervention, language support

6. Dental health care

7. Nutrition, exercise, and addiction

8. Cross-cutting task: strengthening health literacy

9. Cross-cutting task: preventing violence

The Hamburg Institute of Medical Sociology provided scientific support for this process of developing, testing, and implementing a systematic concept of action or a prevention program for a disadvantaged neighborhood as part of Federal Ministry of Research-funded prevention research.

In the following, individual methods and approaches will be presented for the activation and participation of actors and residents in the Lenzsiedlung that have been tested within the framework of collaborations between science and practice, though it must be said, in qualification, that the procedures and methods used mainly served to generate information and gain knowledge in the research process, but, as an important "side" aspect that should not be underestimated, always necessarily also involved the activation and participation of the particular groups of people surveyed.

The following two examples, the "Expert survey" and "Resident survey," are to be seen against this background. The third example reports on successful participation culture in the context of capacity building and development for the implementation and dynamic further development of the prevention program through the "round table" in the Lenzsiedlung.

4. Examples of activation and participation in the Lenzsiedlung

Participatory approaches in community-based health promotion always include techniques and methods of activation and participation in equal measure, as basic elements, and are always also aimed at the main actors in question and the inhabitants of the community, district, or neighborhood. "Participatory" then means that not only the citizens or residents are to be involved in the events and to help shape them, but also, and especially, the professional actors in the field in question. This consideration is taken into account in the following presentation and discussion of methods of community-based health promotion taking place in the Lenzsiedlung in Hamburg-Eimsbüttel. The first section represents the participation of local actors but is only briefly examined because the procedure has already been described in more detail elsewhere [12–15]. The second section concerns the participation of residents through focus groups as well as a (quantitative) survey. In these examples, the focus is on determining the development of capacities in the district. The third section focuses on the direct involvement of citizens in health promotion activities. In the fourth section, the "Lenzgesund" round table is outlined, that is, the collaborative committee on which local professional actors and residents together control the development of the practical project (with the support of research).

4.1 Survey of actors concerning capacity building in the neighborhood

With the help of a survey tool developed by the project, central actors from the health and social sector were asked about capacity building in the district. Capacity building has barely been used as a concept in Germany thus far. Nevertheless, capacity building has been explicitly listed for several years as a benefit dimension and intermediate target parameter for prevention and health promotion. This relatively new indicator – which is still defined to differing degrees of broadness in the literature – essentially refers to:

- the willingness and ability of institutions or professions to develop appropriate structures to be able to successfully offer and maintain a specific action
- the use and mobilization of appropriate resources and collaborative structures; and
- the development of adequate strategies for the implementation and evaluation of measures.
- The questionnaire developed by our team on "capacity building in the district" (Kapazitätsentwicklung im Quartier = KEQ) comprises five thematic complexes or dimensions, which were operationalized with 54 closed items (5-point scales):
- Public participation (level of civic participation, self-initiative of residents, promotion of civic participation)
- Local leadership responsibilities (extent of local leadership, social, and governance skills)
- Available resources (material resources, knowledge and information, social resources)
- Networking and cooperation (local and supra-local networking and collaboration, quality of networking and collaboration)
- Health Promotion (representing the existence and use of health-related infrastructure).

The first pilot study was conducted in June 2006. In addition to the assessment of the current situation (T1), a retrospective assessment of the situation was also to be made before the introduction of individual health promotion offers in May 2001 (T0). In addition to the level of approval, qualitative information was also requested to explain why the statements were judged to be of more or less relevance. Based on a list that was drawn up together with our practice partners, we called on 48 professional actors from the health and social sector (including district development, community work, education, and upbringing) from the area surrounding the Lenzsiedlung to participate in the survey. After sending or handing over the survey documents, only 27 questionnaires were actually evaluated (56% response rate) due to subsequent cancelations and/or short-term unavailability. The attempt to include socially engaged residents in the quantitative study with the same questionnaire was impractical because of the low level of participation; however, we have organized the residents' participation in this issue with different approaches (– > 4.2).

In the following, the results for the five dimensions of capacity development at 3 points in time are summarized in a spider diagram (see **Figure 1**). The average scores are shown per dimension in 2001 and 2006, as well as for the T2 survey in 2008, and, in each case, they can range from 1 to 5 (= best score). The overall positive results for district development and health promotion in the district are to be emphasized: we attribute these, above all, to the general climate of engagement for the neighborhood as well as to the strong commitment and perseverance of individual actors from the health and social sector. There are also positive developments in the field of public involvement – understood as participating or sharing in the community life of the Lenz settlement (e.g., attending information events or neighborhood festivals, using public services). Many respondents attribute this to the more open "climate" in the district, which has been fostered most notably by the use of various activation techniques (e.g., resident surveys, information afternoons), as well as awards and accolades for the district management and the population. However, only partial progress is noted in self-selected initiatives and the assumption of more personal responsibility (primarily in the low-threshold area, such as childcare/fixed preparation).

However, the T2 survey in June 2008, still shows a certain growth or consistency of the values on the spider diagram, which means that, after the seven-year activity phase, stable capacity building and sustainable capacity development in the Lenz estate could be assumed.

All changes T0–T1 and T0–T2 are very pronounced ($ES \geq 0.8$) and highly significant ($p < 0.001$). From T1 to T2, no statistically significant improvements can be detected, but only tendential ones.

Originally called "(Supporting residents through) health care services".

Representation as a spider diagram proved to be particularly suitable for visualizing the results and discussing them with the inhabitants.

However, it must be pointed out that the extent of capacity building is assessed here by the responsible actors themselves, and, so, there is a risk of subjective

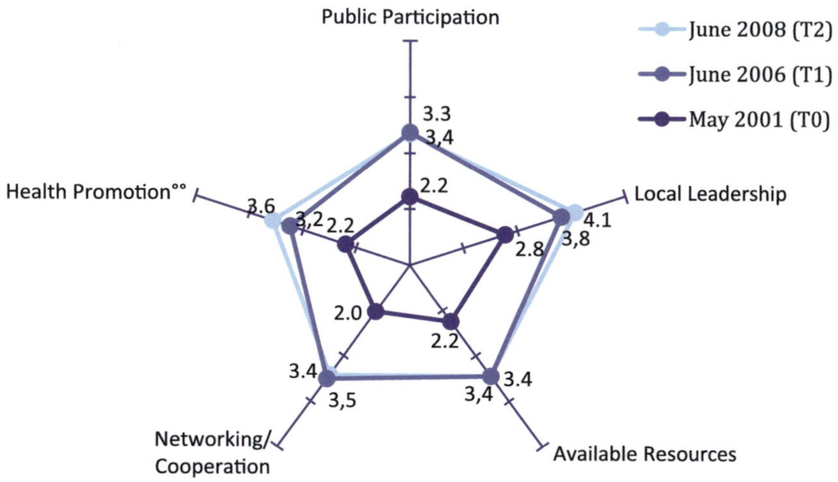

Figure 1.
An overview of the capacity development dimensions (mean values: 1 = worst, 5 = best value) (own illustration).

distortion. For this reason, we also consulted the residents about capacity development, with the aim of validating the expert results.

4.2 Two approaches to the resident survey about capacity development in the neighborhood

In a pretest in the winter of 2010/2011, *focus groups* were carried out to involve the population. The objectives were:

- to triangulate results from previous expert surveys
- to further involve residents and attain information about how they perceive things
- to gain feedback on the "Lenzgesund" prevention program; and – fundamentally associated with the implementation of the focus groups
- to activate residents.

The focus groups consisted of several engaged residents of the Lenzsiedlung who had been selected and who initially worked through a discussion guide as an introduction. In a later step, individual items from the KEQ questionnaire were then discussed.

In addition to the focus groups a *citizen survey (n = 157)* was carried out in the Lenzsiedlung in autumn 2009. This was carried out not by us, but in collaboration with us by the provider of children's and youth services "Lenzsiedlung e.V.," and we were able to introduce some of the same items in the survey as in the KEQ questionnaire and compare them with the results from the focus groups.

It was interesting that the results of the focus groups and the quantitative survey of the population by Lenzsiedlung e.V. were sometimes almost identical. In general, the two surveys of the residents were not completely consistent with the expert judgments, and also differed from each other in some respects.

However, the most important aspect of all three approaches to measuring capacity development was reporting the results. On the one hand, this element of participation was implemented as part of events that were announced and held in the district. On the other hand – more importantly – the results were introduced and discussed at the "Lenzgesund" round table meetings in order to further develop individual fields of action or drive forward strategic planning for the program as a whole.

4.3 Involve and activate residents through a resident survey

The aim of the activating resident survey conducted by our project at the beginning of 2006 was to determine how citizens perceive, use and assess ongoing health promotion and prevention activities in the district, as well as which activities they could possibly participate in themselves or which they could reinitiate themselves. In addition, starting points for future projects were to be identified, and direct participation was sought. We, therefore, once again applied a classic tool in civic involvement, the activating survey.

Two-thirds of the interviews were conducted by means of surveying passers-by. In order to reach migrants with insufficient knowledge of German, about a third of the interviews were conducted by committed residents of the Lenzsiedlung, who interviewed their friends, relatives, and neighbors. Some of these interviews were conducted in Turkish, Farsi, or Urdu. A total of 157 people between the ages of 14 and 58 were interviewed. Due to the survey method, the survey is not representative but provides relevant insights into the views of the population. Selected results of the survey will be presented in brief below.

The existing services were relatively well-known to the respondents; on average, each resident was familiar with about five of the 15 services. The ratings were almost consistently "good" to "very good" (90%). Only for a few services was there a greater number of "moderate" or "bad" reviews.

In addition to the acceptance of the services, the barriers to use perceived by the residents were also of interest. As shown in **Figure 2**, it was deficient information that was most often assumed to be a barrier (40%). Disinterest and a lack of motivation were conjectured by almost a third (31%) of residents and a lack of time by another fifth (19%). An uncertain environment or lack of a sense of belonging playing a role was reported by 12% of respondents. Answers such as "Isolation," "Mistrust" or "Is not the best area" went into this category. Language was conjectured as a barrier by 6%, while lack of money and poor (spatial) accessibility both played a subordinate role, with only two mentions each.

In order to determine what wishes the residents have for health promotion in the district, they were first asked which services they would like to see set up next. The most desired offers were "cooking courses for healthy eating," "addiction counseling," and "smoking cessation" as well as "psychological counseling" (44–37% of respondents).

Another question dealt with the willingness of the respondents to participate, which was answered by 144 of the 157 respondents. Of these, 40% stated that they could imagine actively participating in health-promoting offers. The latter clearly showed that there is great interest among the residents in getting involved and in co-creation. However, the actual participation (even at the presentation of the results) lagged significantly behind the expressed interest.

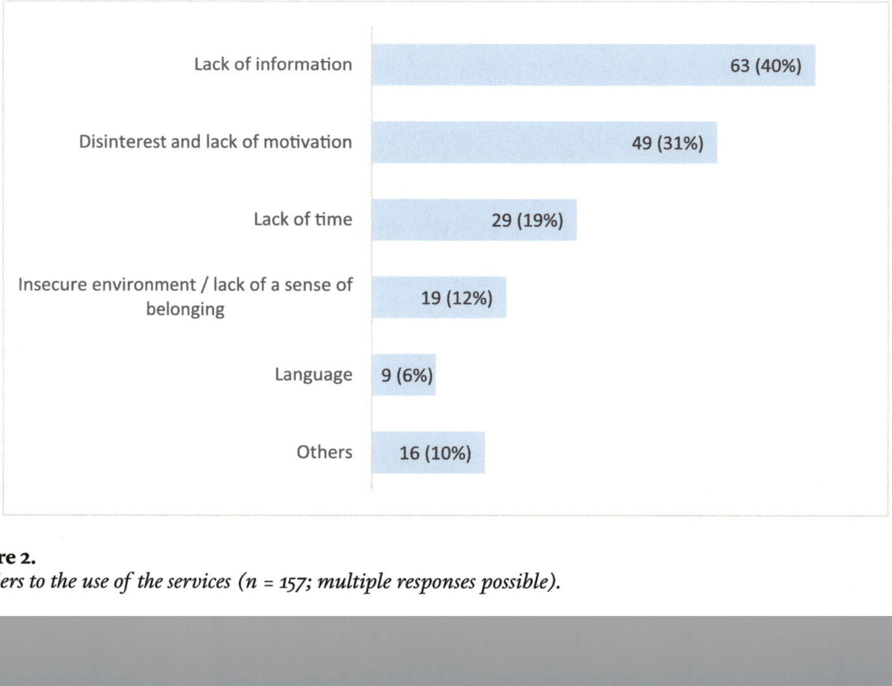

Figure 2.
Barriers to the use of the services (n = 157; multiple responses possible).

4.4 "Lenzgesund" round table participation structure

Round table – this is a metaphor intended to make it clear that no one can sit at the head of the table. Nobody is in charge. Decisions are made together. The "Lenzgesund" round table was held for the first time in autumn 2003 at the initiative of the Eimsbüttel health office in the Lenzsiedlung. It serves as an interface between the actors and the population and aims to establish health promotion and prevention with participation as an area of activity within the district development. Further overarching objectives of the health-promoting activities of the "Lenzgesund" round table are described in detail [16]:

- Providing information and knowledge about health care
- Encouraging motivation to follow a healthy lifestyle
- Activating the population and
- a particularly important concern – connecting the professional actors in the health and social sectors toward more informed and committed collaboration in everyday life and in the implementation of the prevention program.

At its first meetings, the round table more often organized small groups for special tasks, but there were no long-term working groups that were also active between the plenary sessions. Measures and projects were organized by and between individual institutions – in particular, the health office and the Lenzsiedlung Association.

The participation of the residents was envisaged in this initial conception of the round table. However, it became clear that the sessions were not interesting for them, as a collaboration between actors and institutions with regard to the implementation of health promotion and prevention services was becoming more and more important. Therefore, the development of professional concepts and professional decision-making processes mainly determined the discussion at the round table. In addition to the function of ensuring information exchange, the round table thus increasingly had the function of an advisory body.

The adoption of the Lenzgesund prevention program in January 2005 strengthened the structure of the round table as a result of the determination of objectives or fields of action and the establishment of permanent working groups. In June 2011, 10 to 12 institutions with 14 to 18 representatives formed the fixed core of the round table; others were only present occasionally (see **Figure 3**).

The "Lenzgesund" round table has significantly promoted networking among actors and their areas of activity, and thus the implementation of the prevention program. However, from the point of view of our practice partner, the Hamburg-Eimsbüttel Health Office, it cannot be expected to provide permanent and continuous monitoring and implementation for the program. It is more of an instrument of ideation and activation.

The experience of recent years shows that it is possible to activate a relatively large number of institutions and their representatives to exchange information and ideas. However, for many participants, this purpose was not sufficient for a permanent, regular engagement. Even so, there was a smaller group that was continuously involved. In addition, communication at the round table has developed into a series of sustainable working relationships in everyday life.

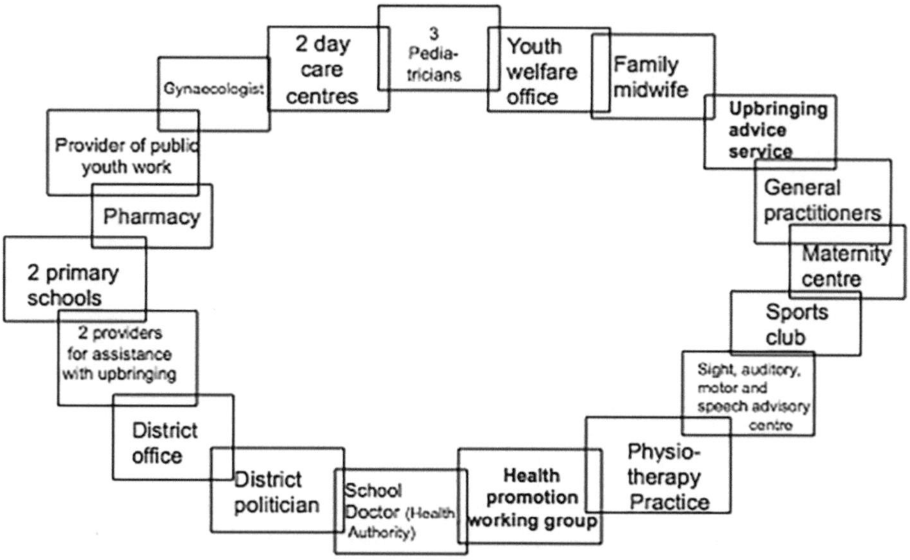

Figure 3.
Facilities at the "Lenzgesund" round table.

For the health office as the organizer of the "Lenzgesund" prevention program, this meant that, in addition to the networking committee, the "Lenzgesund" round table, it needed stable working alliances with other individual institutions. Such alliances developed with the "Lenzsiedlung" Association and in approaches with the "Rauhen Haus", a further free provider of active social work in the district. The aim was also to strengthen collaborations with schools in the area surrounding the Lenzsiedlung.

Interesting information on the performance of the task and the role of the round table is gained from a survey of the participants. According to the respondents, the round table particularly fulfills the tasks of exchanging information, identifying problem areas, and developing goals, as well as the general management and further development of the prevention program (values 3.8–4.0 on a five-point scale, with the best value being 5).

In addition, the district diagnoses published as part of the research projects are considered important for the implementation of prevention and health promotion in the Lenzsiedlung [16, 17] and were made available and discussed at the round table, as they can be used to "provide better and targeted support."

The importance of the round table was also assessed in the context of a further survey in the autumn of 2008, with the instrument for measuring KEQ already presented. Here, too, it can be seen that, compared to other networking structures in and around the district, the importance of the "Lenzgesund" round table in the area is evaluated as important to very important, i.e., it holds an outstanding position.

From our point of view, it can be said that the "Lenzgesund" round table, with its continuous and regular work, played an informative, orienting, motivating, moderating, and coordinating role. Unfortunately, the original intention to involve the residents directly in the meetings of the round table could not be realized because there were not enough interested residents to take part continuously.

The participatory approaches and project experiences presented in the community-based health promotion activities show the diverse possibilities of setting-related involvement and activation of actors and residents [18] using the example of the Lenzsiedlung.

5. Discussion

Participation can be realized to different degrees depending on the practical conditions within a health promotion program and the living conditions of the target group. The object is to find the appropriate level of participation based on the conditions [5].

This text presents examples of participation and involvement of key implementation actors as well as parts of the population of a disadvantaged neighborhood. Both the surveying of the main actors and the surveying of the population represented a complex approach of activating and involving different groups, following a systematic and complex procedure. For this, the corresponding resources must be to hand and available, as can certainly be the case in a project between science and practice. This was different with the "Lenzgesund" round table participatory mode also presented – which can also be designed and implemented within the framework of the standard tasks.

If one wants to classify the examples in the step models, one may say that the presented forms of surveys – in simplified terms – are about "being allowed to have a say." In the model (**Figure 4**) they are to be classified as medium-to-high participatory approaches, all the way up to "partnership-based collaboration." They do not

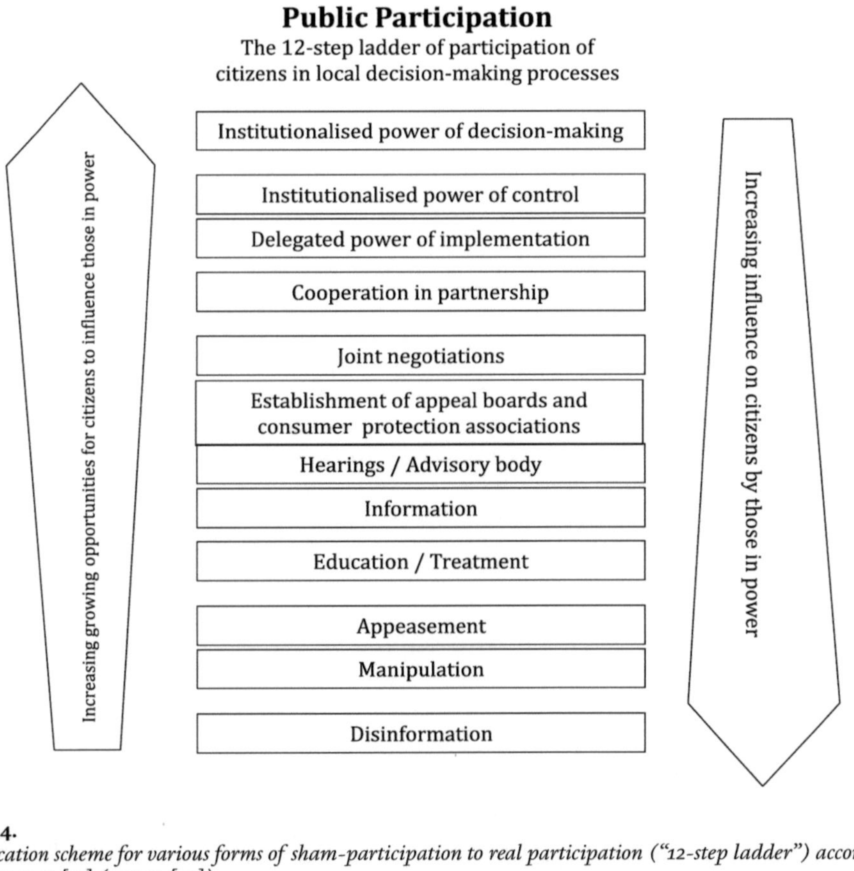

Figure 4.
Classification scheme for various forms of sham-participation to real participation ("12-step ladder") according to Trojan 2001 [19] (source: [20]).

reach the range of categories for which decision-making power must be handed over to the residents. The round table is also not a body endowed with authority and decision-making powers that decides on the services to be provided by other actors, institutions, or bodies. In the language of the ladder models, the round table is a partnership-based collaboration in the interests of consultation, involvement, networking, and voluntary prioritization by participating institutions for their health-related activities in this disadvantaged settlement.

Looking at the capacity-building process in its entirety and over time, the Lenzsiedlung saw a relatively large amount of civic involvement and social participation on a small scale at different levels, for example, the health talks for women, the many neighborhood festivals and meet-up initiatives, which were repeatedly awarded prizes for best neighborhood. If we take a look at the different traditional and creative participatory instruments, methods, and procedures mentioned at the start, it becomes clear that these usually fit with programs and (standard) activities that are equipped with special and sometimes considerable resources for participation and civic involvement. The possible participatory methods are, in each case, always strongly contextual, i.e., dependent on financial resources, the subject matter, the nature of the program, and, not least, the competence encountered among the citizens to be involved.

6. Conclusions

Civic involvement seems to be particularly pronounced when no very big decisions have to be made. For this context, there is a wealth of techniques and procedures that can be unpacked from the method tool kit. However, this idea of "always just being asked" (and, unfortunately, often without any consequences) does not necessarily promote participation in the long run.

A successful example of participation in terms of more concrete, manageable decisions include (in Germany, but similarly also in other countries) financial disposal funds, e.g., in the context of social district development. Here, the inhabitants of disadvantaged districts and neighborhoods can co-decide which money can be spent for what and, above all, how quickly and unbureaucratically this can be done (e.g., in the design of building entrances). This is where the particular success of this model lies. This example also shows that it is not so much a fundamental question of power that motivates those involved but, rather, the unbureaucratic implementation of participatory programming.

According to the Ottawa Charter and the actors and scientists who refer to it, civic involvement and participation are considered normative "must have" in community-based health promotion and prevention. No objection can be made to this normative requirement. It is simply that participation should not be elevated from norm to dogma. Not everything that comes from the top is bad just because it comes from the top (see, for example, the programs of urban social development!). Furthermore, participation must not become an end in itself, in the sense that it is practiced but has no consequences. This can then lead to frustration and disappointment and destroy the confidence that has already been built up. It is quite fatal if procedures and methods of participation can ultimately be turned against those involved, with the result that, under the guise of quasi-democratic legitimation, interests can be enforced that a majority of the citizens involved do not have.

7. Way forward

Of course, offers, and procedures for involvement and participation are generally positive, since they are already legitimate for democratic reasons alone. They should be implemented in health care regardless of whether there is empirical evidence on their effectiveness in managing disease and maintaining health.

Certainly, not all potential and possibilities of involvement and participation on the part of the population or the target group(s) were exploited in the implementation of the "Lenzgesund" prevention program. Participation and involvement naturally require professional management for their diverse procedures and forms in program development and implementation. At this point, however, the main actors already overloaded by the standard tasks are often overwhelmed from a technical and time perspective. In order to prevent nonuse, under-use, and misuse, it would be necessary to have municipal health promotion management that explicitly provides for the organization and implementation of civic involvement in the job description and also makes the necessary resources available for this purpose.

Acknowledgements

We would like to thank our colleagues Waldemar Süß and Karin Wolf (formerly Mossakowski) for the dedicated research work they have carried out over the many years of our three joint projects!

We thank the (former) Federal Ministry of Education and Research (BMBF) for funding the three projects:

1. BMBF research project "Capacity building for prevention and health promotion among children and parents in a disadvantaged neighborhood" (FKZ: 01 EL 0414), 2005–2008.

2. BMBF research project "Long-term evaluation and transfer potential of the" Lenzgesund "prevention program – development of practical aids for interventions, evaluation and monitoring of participatory health promotion in disadvantaged neighborhoods" (FKZ: 01 EL 0812), 2009–2012.

BMBF research project "Long-term evaluation of complex interventions in neighborhood-related health promotion and prevention measures – An investigation of community capacities ten years after the start of the Lenzgesund program" (FKZ: 01 EL 1410), 2014–2017.

Last but not least, we would like to thank the institutions, actors and residents of the Lenzsiedlung for their dedicated work toward the program's practical implementation and during the accompanying research!

Conflicts of interest

The authors declare no conflict of interest.

Author details

Alf Trojan*, Christian Lorentz and Stefan Nickel
Institute of Medical Sociology, University Medical Center Hamburg-Eppendorf, Hamburg, Germany

*Address all correspondence to: trojan@uke.de

References

[1] Ottawa Charta für Gesundheitsförderung, Weltgesundheitsorganisation (WHO). Ottawa-Charta zur Gesundheitsförderung. Kopenhagen: WHO-Regionalbüro für Europa; 1986. Available from: https://www.who.int/teams/health-promotion/enhanced-well-being/first-global-conference [Accessed: April 2, 2013]

[2] Wright MT, editor. Partizipative Qualitätsentwicklung in der Gesundheitsförderung und Prävention. Bern: Verlag Hans Huber; 2010

[3] Laverack G, editor. Gesundheitsförderung und Empowerment. In: Grundlagen und Methoden mit vielen Beispielen aus der praktischen Arbeit. Gamburg: Verlag für Gesundheitsförderung; 2010

[4] Loss J, Eichhorn C, Gehlert J, Donhauser J, Wise M, Nagel E. Gemeindenahe Gesundheitsförderung - Herausforderung an die Evaluation. Gesundheitswesen. 2007;**69**:77-87

[5] Wright MT, Block M, von Unger H. Stufen der Partizipation in der Gesundheitsförderung. Ein Modell zur Beurteilung von Beteiligung. Infodienst für Gesundheitsförderung. 2007;**3**:4-5

[6] Callahan K. Citizen participation: Models and methods. International Journal of Public Administration. 2007;**30**(11):1179-1196

[7] Penta L. Community Organizing. Hamburg: Menschen verändern ihre Stadt. edition körber stiftung; 2007

[8] ICPHR – International Collaboration for Participatory Health Research. Position Paper 1: What Is Participatory Health Research? Version: May 2013. Berlin: International Collaboration for Participatory Health Research; 2013

[9] Wallerstein N, Duran B, Oetzel J, Minkler M. Community-Based Participatory Research for Health: Advancing Social and Health Equity. San Francisco: Jossey-Bass; 2018

[10] Wright MT, Kongats K. Participatory Health Research: Voices from around the World. New York: Springer; 2018

[11] Zinser C. Aktivierung und Beteiligung von Familien. München: Deutsches Jugendinstitut e.V; 2004

[12] Trojan A, Nickel S. Zur Messung von Kapazitätsentwicklung im Quartier. In: Kolip P, Müller V, editors. Qualität von Gesundheitsförderung und Prävention. Bern: Verlag Hans Huber; 2009

[13] Labonte R, Laverack G. Capacity building in health promotion, part 2: Whose use? And with what measurement? Critical Public Health. 2001;**2**:129-138

[14] Goodman RM, Speers MA, Mcleroy K, Fawcett S, Kegler M, Parker E, et al. Identifying and defining the dimensions of community capacity to provide a basis for measurement. Health Educational & Behavior. 1998;**3**:258-278

[15] Trojan A. Lenzgesund – A long-term community health promotion programme in a deprived neighborhood and its evaluation. In: Mollaoğlu M, editor. Health Promotion. 2022. pp. S.31-S.40. DOI: 10.5772/intechopen.101913 [Accessed: January 1, 2022]

[16] Mossakowski K, Nickel S, Schäfer I, Süß W, Trojan A, Werner S.

Quartiersdiagnose Lenzgesund - mehr Gesundheit ins Quartier! Hamburg: Daten und Ansätze zur Gesundheitsförderung in der Lenzsiedlung in Hamburg-Eimsbüttel; 2006

[17] Kohler S, Mossakowski K, Süß W, Nickel S, Trojan A. Beiträge zur Quartiersdiagnose - Kindergesundheit in der Lenzsiedlung. Hamburg; 2007

[18] Mossakowski K, Süß W, Trojan A. Partizipative Ansätze in der gemeindenahen Gesundheitsförderung, Stufen der Partizipation und Beispiel aus einem Wissenschaftspraxisprojekt in der Hamburger Lenzsiedlung. In: Prävention und Gesundheitsförderung. Vol. Heft 3. Heidelberg: Springer Verlag; 2009

[19] Trojan A. In: Trojan A, Legewie H, editors. Bürgerbeteiligung - Die 12-stufige Leiter der Beteiligung von Bürgern an lokalen Entscheidungsprozessen. Vol. 324. Verlag für Akademische Schriften, Frankfurt am Main: Nachhaltige Gesundheit und Entwicklung; 2001

[20] Wright MT. Partizipation: Mitentscheidung der Bürgerinnen und Bürger. In: Bundeszentrale für gesundheitliche Aufklärung (BZgA) (Hrsg.), Leitbegriffe der Gesundheitsförderung und Prävention. Strategien und Methoden: Glossar zu Konzepten; 2020. DOI: 10.17623/BZGA:224-i084-1.0 [Accessed: April 2, 2023]

Section 2

Approaches to Health Promotion

Chapter 4

Causal Structure for the Healthy Longevity Based on the Socioeconomic Status, Healthy Diet and Lifestyle, and Three Health Dimensions, in Japan

Tanji Hoshi

Abstract

This chapter aims to clarify the causal relationship between healthy life expectancy, socioeconomic status, dietary habits, lifestyle habits, and three health factors, as indicated by the WHO. In addition, the annual income threshold for couples to maintain a certain number of survival days will be clarified. Of the 16,462 elderly people aged 65 and over, 13,195 were included in the self-assessment questionnaire survey conducted in September 2001. A follow-up survey was completed in 2004, and 8,162 survivors were followed until August 2007. From a cross-lagged effects variation model, causal relationships were analyzed using longitudinal survival days between 2004 and 2007. After estimating a best-fit model, we discovered that current dietary and lifestyle habits did not determine healthy longevity. However, the survival days were more directly affected by three health-related dimensions three years earlier based on educational attainment and previous annual income indirectly. This study suggests that it might be of great importance for elderly individuals to emphasize income maintenance rather than focusing on diet and lifestyle improvements. In addition to showing a statistically significant relationship between income and survival days, we clarified that there is a threshold for income to maintain a certain number of survival days. For the elderly, it was 4.5 million yen(3,462 US $) for both sexes as a marital yearly income.

Keywords: survival rate, life style, socioeconomic status, income threshold, aged, Japan

1. Introduction

The increase in life expectancy of Japanese people is well-known worldwide [1]. Many studies have investigated the factors that determine the life expectancy of Japanese people [2]. In 2019, men had a life expectancy of 80.41, while healthy life expectancy was 72.68, a difference of 8.73 years. The average life expectancy of women was 86.44 years, and the healthy life expectancy was 75.38 years, with a range of 12.06 years (Ministry of Health, Labor and Welfare 2022) [3].

In recent years, attention has been paid to the determinants regarding the average life expectancy and healthy life expectancy of older Japanese people. However, most of these studies used cross-sectional and ecological data [4, 5]. Therefore, it has been complicated and unclear to comprehensively analyze the causal structure, and various factors, including socioeconomic factors, for the healthy life expectancy of older people over their lifetime.

Canada's Lalonde Report [6] and USA Healthy People Strategy [7] addressed the importance of lifestyle habits related to diet and health, against the background that the contribution to medical health has not been significant to date. Many studies have explained the health effects of certain lifestyles [8, 9].

A favorable lifestyle reduces early mortality in people with specific diseases and lifestyles [10, 11]. In a large cohort of Japanese people, Tamakoshi et al. [12] showed that lifestyle significantly impacted life expectancy. However, lifestyle is not the only factor associated with individual survival days. Socioeconomic factors and the three health factors indicated by the WHO, physical and mental, and social factors, should also be considered.

Several reports highlight the impact of socioeconomic status on life expectancy. Socioeconomic differences were significantly associated with life expectancy [13, 14] and survival in older people [15]. Sugiura et al. [16] reported socioeconomic status as a background to the rapid increase in life expectancy of Japanese people after World War II. Considering the impact of Japan's socioeconomic position on health, Kagamori et al. [17] concluded that the difference in mortality was not trivial. However, research results have not been presented on the direct and indirect causal structure of socioeconomic conditions and life expectancy.

The World Health Organization (WHO) defines health as follows: Health is a better physical, mental, and social well-being, not merely the absence of illness or infirmity [18]. Based on this definition, studies have reported that three health-related aspects of physical, mental, and social well-being are related to life expectancy [19–24], Specifically, physical activity and function [19, 20], cognitive vulnerability and self-rated health [21–23], and social connections [24] are statistically significantly related to survival in older adults. However, except for a few studies [25, 26], no studies have clarified causal structures associated with three health aspects, survival and socioeconomic status.

The fundamental hypothesis model is shown in **Figure 1**. This model indicates that healthy survival days and not-bedridden status would be determined by healthy dietary and lifestyle habits and three health-related dimensions based on socioeconomic status as a structural and causal relationship.

Therefore, the objectives of this chapter were to clarify the causal relationships among healthy dietary and lifestyle habits, socioeconomic status, and three health-related dimensions related to healthy longevity among Japanese elderly suburban dwellers. Covariance structure analysis clarified how large and causally each latent variable shown in **Figure 1** has a causal relationship with healthy longevity, a latent dependent variable.

It has become clear that it is essential to live satisfactorily in terms of health and the amount of annual income influenced by individual educational background.

What is the income threshold required to maintain survival? The relationship between per capita national product and average life expectancy for each country and its income threshold for longevity are reported. Here, a connection is shown in which

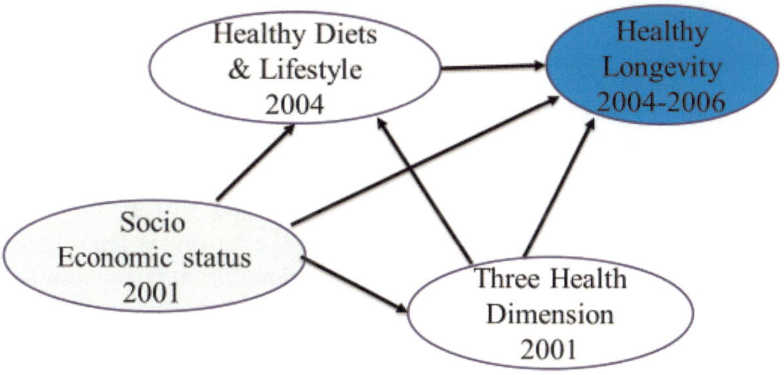

Figure 1.
Causal structural relationships to the healthy longevity as a hypothesis model.

the higher the per capita national product of a country, the longer the average life expectancy. When it exceeded more than 4.500 US $, almost no extension of life expectancy was seen, and it occupied a practically constant level [27].

Costa Rica's average life expectancy, which is less than 10% of the per capita national product of the United States of America, was almost at the same level as that of the United States. In this way, along with the relationship between the value of national production and average life expectancy, the national product threshold has been clarified to ensure a certain average life expectancy [27].

However, no studies have been reported that clarify the annual income on an individual basis and the income threshold for maintaining a certain number of survival days, except in the six-year follow-up studies in urban suburbs and areas reported by the authors [25, 26].

Therefore, in this study, we will discuss the relationship between marital annual income and survival days in older people living at home in urban suburbs, citing a part of a previous study that also aimed to clarify the family yearly income threshold to ensure a certain number of survival days.

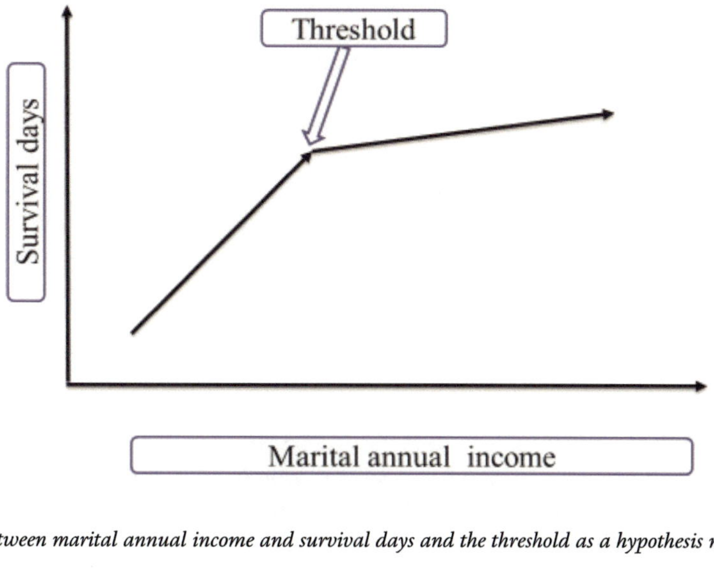

Figure 2.
Relationship between marital annual income and survival days and the threshold as a hypothesis model.

In the case of achieving the research purpose, the support method by health education specialists who support health is expected to be linked to new health support based on the process of taking into account the significance of the underlying income and enabling people to live positively against the background of a certain income, and as a result, specific desirable lifestyle habit might be maintained.

In addition to the significance of income, which is particularly important as a socioeconomic factor, it is expected that scientific income criteria regarding how much income can be used to maintain a certain level of survival can be presented.

We hypothesized that there is a significant relationship between annual marital income and survival days and that there is a threshold in this association. The hypothetical model is shown in **Figure 2**.

However, no studies have been reported that clarify the annual income on an individual basis and the income threshold for maintaining a certain number of survival days, except in the six-year follow-up studies in urban suburbs and areas reported by the authors [25].

2. Methods

2.1 Participants and study setting

Details of the survey method were shown in previous studies [25, 26]. Here, only the main survey methods are shown.

In September 2001, we surveyed all elderly people (65 years and older) living in their homes in a municipality near Tokyo. Of the 16,462 participants, 13,195 (80.2% of respondents) gave informed consent to participate in the study and returned a self-administered questionnaire by mail. A second questionnaire was mailed to respondents in September 2004. As a result, 8,558 people responded. There were 505 relocations, 914 deaths, and 3218 no responses. The survey respondents were all elderly people living in their homes over 65. We tracked all participants until August 31, 2007, and obtained personal data using IDs for 8,162 deaths and survivals through the City Hall Resident Registry.

The municipalities studied are urban suburbs that partially developed as suburban cities from the 1970s to the 1990s, including the period of high economic growth, to accommodate the increase in workers and their families in the metropolitan area. The total population of the cities surveyed was about 140,000 as of 2001, and 9.6% of the population was over 65 years old, almost half of the national average (17.3%) in 2000.

2.2 Observed measurement variables

Many observed variables and latent variables were used to clarify the causal structure using different factors in the survey year. The latent variables were determined by exploratory factor analysis, as shown in section 3.2. The question methods, options, and survey methods of the observed variables used in the survey are shown in the literature of previous studies [25, 26].

Socioeconomic status in 2001 was assessed via educational attainment and annual income. Levels of educational attainment were categorized into four groups; graduation from junior high school, graduation from high school, those achieving a higher academic level than junior college, and those who did not want to respond. Annual income levels fell into four categories; less than one million Japanese yen(equivalent to less than US $7,400), less than three million yen, less than five million yen, and more than seven million yen in 2001.

Healthy dietary and lifestyle habits in 2004 were assessed by the dietary health score and the healthy lifestyle score, respectively [25, 26]. The three health-related dimensions examined in our study consisted of physical, mental, and social health components [25, 26].

2.3 Analyses

Detailed analysis of analytical methods, methods, and fitness was described in previous studies [25, 26]. Respondents aged 80 and older and those with more than a moderate degree of long-term care in the 2001 survey were excluded from the analyses due to an increased and indispensable deviation in their measurement variables. All data obtained were evaluated by degree to examine differences between males and females using Kendall's tau rank correlation coefficient. Exploratory factor analysis was used to fit all observed variables to corresponding latent variables.

The most important research method of this research is structural equation modeling (SEM). The analysis software used AMOS ver.28 for Windows (IBM). The analysis data used longitudinal follow-up data over seven years. Based on data from the 2001 survey, the 2004 survey investigated the three factors of a healthy diet, lifestyle, and health, as well as the degree of care required. We also clarified the number of days lived from 2004 to 2007. For causal structures, we used all combinations of four latent variables to find the model with the best fit.

Estimating the best-fitting model was carried out by the maximum likelihood method of SEM. The optimization algorithm was implemented with no-missing-data parameters. The direct, indirect, and total standardized effects of different latent variables on the endogenous health and life condition variable were measured by gender. The models employed indices criteria for assessing model fitness. Goodness-of-fit was approved by the chi-square goodness-of-fit test ($\chi 2$, degree of freedom, P value), NFI (Normed fit index), 1FI (Incremental fit index), RMSEA (Root mean square error of approximation) for the structural relationship model. Results were considered statistically significant if the p-value was less than 0.05.

A mutual agreement was signed between the city and local governments and Tokyo Metropolitan University regarding protecting individual privacy during the entire survey process. In this agreement, the confidentiality obligation was confirmed, and personal information handled by the university was limited to IDs. In September 2004 and September 2007, consent was obtained from the Tokyo Metropolitan University Graduate School Ethics Committee for a follow-up survey on manufacturing.

3. Results

3.1 Measurement variables

Of 8,162 eligible participants, included in the analysis were 7,066 individuals (male, 3,409; female, 3,657) aged lower than 80 years and with either no long-term care or the mildest degree of long-term care utilized in September 2001.

Previous studies detailed the critical results of the observed variables [25, 26]. The mean survival days between September 1, 2004, and August 31, 2007, were fewer in males than in females. 2.3 percent of male and 3.0 percent of female participants had degenerated to either the middle or severest degrees of long-term care in 2004 compared to 2001.

Compared with males, females displayed significantly lower educational attendance and annual income, deemed a gender disparity (Kendall's tau rank correlation coefficients were -0.376, $p < 0.001$ and -0.236, $p < 0.001$, respectively).

Regarding the dietary health score, most participants were distributed below seven points, while in the healthy lifestyle category, most participants scored above two points. The results indicated that many people enjoyed healthy lifestyles, although many later older people had an unhealthy diet.

3.2 Results of exploratory factor analysis

We use the latent variables obtained through exploratory factor analysis for a hypothesized model. Factor 1 indicated high loadings, particularly for self-rated health variables, and displayed a high confidence coefficient. Self-rated health and daily life satisfaction, except for the number of comorbid conditions, were termed "mental health factors" related to the three health-related dimensions. The number of comorbid conditions was a negative factor by itself. It is considered considerably associated with the physical condition since the comorbidities tended to include more common diseases such as hypertension, diabetes, and cardiovascular disease, apart from mental disorders among the target population.

Along with the number of comorbid conditions, BADL and IADL, excluding the frequency of going outside, informed the labeling of factor 2 as "physical health." We emphasized the social aspect of the frequency of going outside over the physical part. Therefore, factor 3 was identified as "social health" and included communication with the neighborhood, hobby-related activities, and frequency of going outside.

Factor 4 was termed "Healthy Dietary and Lifestyle habit" and involved healthy dietary and lifestyle habit variables. Finally, factor 5 was "Socioeconomic Status" and indicated educational attainment and annual income. The cumulative contribution proportion of the above five factors was 40.5 percent.

3.3 Causal relationship "Healthy Dietary and Lifestyle" and "healthy longevity" model

Figure 3 shows the causal relationship between "Healthy Dietary and Lifestyle", and "Healthy Longevity" for both sexes. The models fit the data well with the following fit indices: NFI = 0.995, IFI = 0.997, and RMSEA = 0.008. R-squared values also fit well: 19 percent for males and 13 percent for females.

Based on this model, "Healthy and Longevity" were significantly affected by "Healthy Dietary and Lifestyles" for both sexes significantly. And we observed a relatively significant direct effect of the "Healthy Diet and Lifestyles" on "Healthy Longevity", with a 0.48 standardized path coefficient for males and 0.36 for females. In this model, we are not concerned about socioeconomic status and three health dimensions as confounding factors.

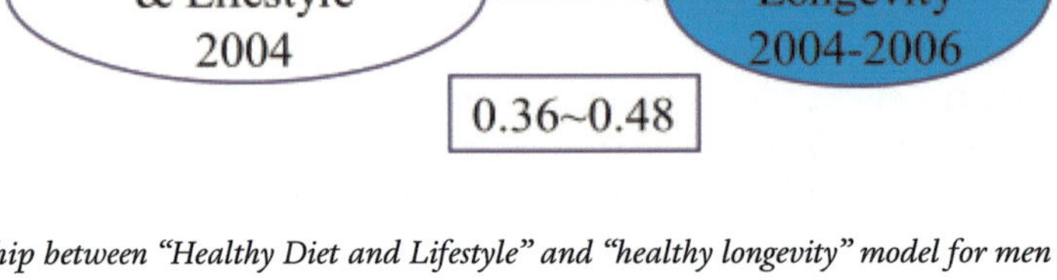

Figure 3.
Causal relationship between "Healthy Diet and Lifestyle" and "healthy longevity" model for men and female.

DOI: http://dx.doi.org/10.5772/intechopen.111910

If only the causal structure of the two latent variables shown in **Figure 3** is analyzed, the more desirable the latent variables of "Healthy diet and Lifestyle." The more desirable the similarly dependent latent variables, the degree of care required. Then, it will be interpreted that "Healthy longevity," a long survival day with a low degree of care needed, becomes statistically significant.

3.4 Structure relationships with "socioeconomic status," "Healthy Diet and Lifestyle," "Three Health-related Dimensions," and "healthy longevity"

We adopted and analyzed the statistically best-fitting models by sex using SEM. **Figure 4** shows the models for male and female participants presenting causal relationships among the latent variables. The models fit the data well with the following fit indices: NFI = 0.861, IFI = 0.872, and RMSEA = 0.025. R-squared values also work well: 81 percent for males and 71 percent for females.

The models depict the pathways from "Socioeconomic Status" in 2001 via "Three Health-related Dimensions" in 2001 and "Healthy Diet and Lifestyle" in 2004, leading to both sexes' "Healthy Longevity" from 2004 to 2006.

In addition, the paths from "Three Health-related Dimensions" approached the "Healthy Diet and Lifestyle." We observed a relatively significant direct effect of the "Three Health-related Dimensions" on "Healthy Longevity," with a 0.90 standardized path coefficient (SPC) for males and 0.84 SPC for females. On the other hand, the direct effect of "Healthy diet and Lifestyle" on "Healthy Longevity" was nearly zero (0.00 ∼ 0.02).

The total effect of "Three Health-related Dimensions" and "Healthy Diet and Lifestyle" supported by "Socioeconomic Status" on "Healthy Longevity" indicated considerably large SPCs for males (0.444) and females (0.580) as a total effect.

3.5 Marital annual income threshold to ensure a certain number of survival days

We used a one-way analysis of variance to analyze the threshold marital annual income to secure a certain number of survival days. A significant difference was tested

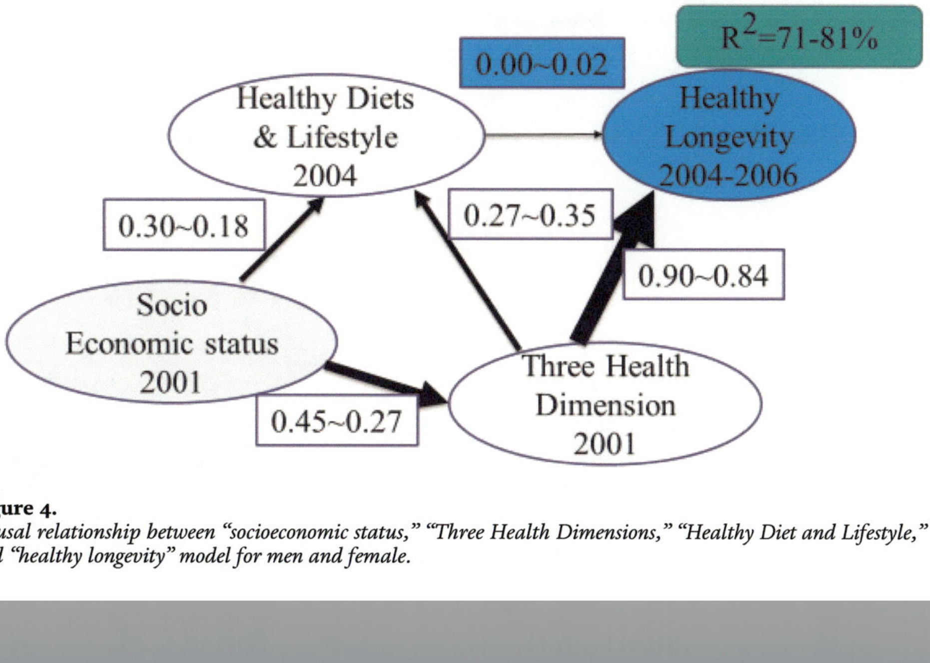

Figure 4.
Causal relationship between "socioeconomic status," "Three Health Dimensions," "Healthy Diet and Lifestyle," and "healthy longevity" model for men and female.

for all combinations of annual income classes by Tamhane's test, which does not assume equal variances [25].

In addition to showing a statistically significant relationship between income and survival days, we clarified that there is a threshold for income to maintain a certain number of survival days.

In the group of 4 million yen or more but less than 5 million yen, there was no significant difference compared to the survival days of the group with more than that. Therefore, 4.5 million yen, the group's median value of 4 million yen to less than 5 million yen, was regarded as the income threshold for maintaining a certain number of survival days (**Table 1**).

The X-axis shown in **Figure 5** is the average income, and the Y-axis indicates the number of days an individual lives. The analysis of older people in suburban cities shows that an income threshold can be seen to ensure a certain number of survival

Sex	(I) Marital annual income	(J) Marital annual income	(I-J)	Standard error	p value	95% Confidential interval	
Men	less than 1 million	less than 2 million	−74.9	47.0	0.917	−218.3	68.4
		less than 3 million	−128.3	44.0	0.078	−262.9	6.3
		less than 4 million	−156.4	43.5	**0.008**	−289.5	−23.3
		less than 5 million	−191.2	44.7	**0.001**	−327.9	−54.5
		more than 7 million	−228.9	44.7	**0.000**	−365.5	−92.3
		more than 7 million	−245.2	44.0	**0.000**	−379.8	−110.6
	less than 2 million	less than 3 million	−53.4	26.6	0.620	−134.1	27.4
		less than 4 million	−81.5	25.7	0.033	−159.7	−3.3
		less than 5 million	−116.3	27.8	**0.001**	−200.6	−32.0
		less than 7 million	−154.0	27.7	**0.000**	−238.2	−69.7
		more than 7 million	−170.3	26.6	**0.000**	−251.1	−89.5
	less than 3 million	less than 4 million	−28.1	19.8	0.972	−88.3	32.0
		less than 5 million	−62.9	22.4	0.100	−130.0	5.0
		less than 7 million	−100.6	22.3	0.000	−168.4	−32.7
		more than 7million	−116.9	20.9	0.000	−180.4	−53.4
	less than 4 million	less than 5 million	−34.8	21.4	0.899	−99.6	30.0
		less than 7 million	−72.5	21.3	0.015	−137.2	−7.7
		more than 7 million	−88.8	19.8	**0.000**	−149.0	−28.6
	less than 5 million	less than 7 million	−37.7	23.7	0.918	−109.7	34.3
		more than 7 million	−54.0	22.4	0.287	−122.0	14.0
	less than 7 million	more than 7 million	−16.3	22.3	1.000	−84.2	51.6
Female	less than 1 million	less than 2 million	−48.1	20.8	0.358	−111.2	15.0
		less than 3 million	−103.5	20.0	**0.000**	−164.3	−42.7
		less than 4 million	−131.8	19.7	**0.000**	−191.6	−72.0
		less than 5 million	−180.7	18.9	**0.000**	−238.1	−123.3

Sex	(I) Marital annual income	(J) Marital annual income	(I-J)	Standard error	p value	95% Confidential interval	
		more than 7 million	−155.0	22.4	**0.000**	−222.9	−87.0
		more than 7 million	−140.9	24.3	**0.000**	−214.6	−67.1
	less than 2 million	less than 3 million	−55.4	16.8	0.021	−106.5	−4.4
		less than 4 million	−83.7	16.4	**0.000**	−133.6	−33.8
		less than 5 million	−132.6	15.5	**0.000**	−179.6	−85.6
		less than 7 million	−106.9	19.6	**0.000**	−166.3	−47.4
		more than 7 million	−92.8	21.7	**0.000**	−158.8	−26.8
	less than 3 million	less than 4 million	−28.3	15.4	0.769	−75.1	18.6
		less than 5 million	−77.2	14.1	**0.000**	−120.9	−33.4
		less than 7 million	−51.5	18.7	0.121	−108.4	5.5
		more than 7 million	−37.3	20.9	0.806	−101.1	26.4
	less than 4 million	less than 5 million	−48.9	14.0	**0.010**	−91.3	−6.5
		less than 7 million	−23.2	18.4	0.992	−79.1	32.7
		more than 7 million	−9.1	20.6	1.000	−71.9	53.8
	less than 5 million	less than 7 million	25.7	17.5	0.960	−27.6	79.1
		more than 7 million	39.8	19.9	0.625	−20.7	100.4
	less than 7 million	more than 7 million	14.1	23.2	1.000	−56.5	84.7

Table 1.
One-way ANOVA of survival days by marital annual income.

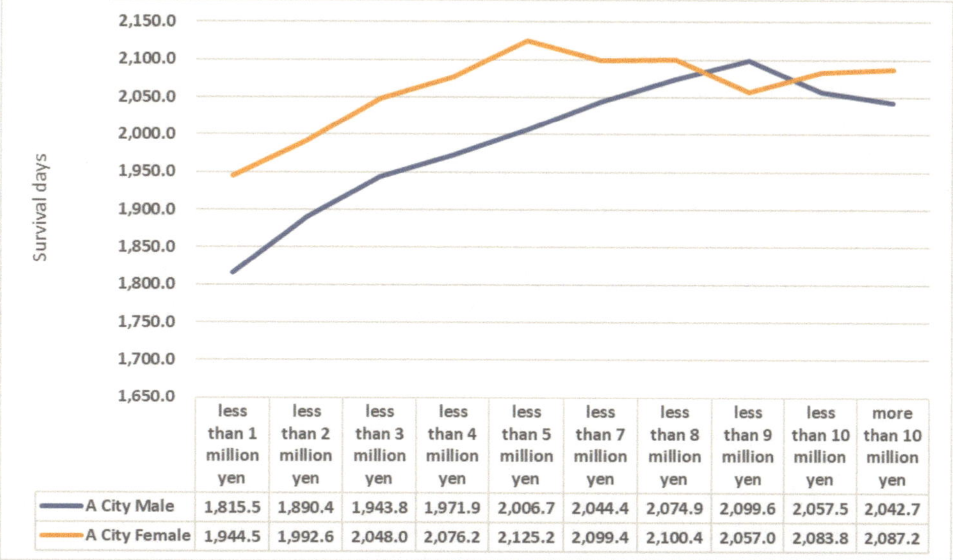

Figure 5.
Annual income threshold for survival days among suburban elderly people for both sexes.

days. These results suggest that older adults living in the suburbs need a certain amount of income to provide a certain number of survival days.

4. Discussion

4.1 Socioeconomic status, dietary and lifestyle habits, three health-related dimensions, and healthy survival days

Until now, a vast amount of health education has been targeted at elderly populations to foster diet and healthy behavioral change attempts. The underlying evidence supported these aims demonstrating that a healthy diet and lifestyle habits improve individual healthy longevity [6–12].

In contrast, our study revealed that current dietary and lifestyle habits did not determine healthy longevity among the suburban Japanese elderly but by the three health-related dimensions observed three years prior and indirectly by their educational attainment and previous annual income.

This original scientific evidence suggests that it might be of great importance for older people to particularly emphasize the maintenance of mental well-being, physical activity, and social communication/participation based on income rather than urging an improvement of their diet or other health-related behaviors.

It should be noted that this unique scientific evidence suggests the need to maintain mental health, physical activity, and social health for older adults to develop desirable diets and lifestyles. At the same time, they suggested that socioeconomic foundations are essential for the three sensual three health dimension.

It might be incorrect to understand that healthy longevity has become due to advantageous lifestyles. Based on our original causal structure analyses, it should be noted that older people with secured income that allows them to have favorable lifestyle habits may have healthy longevity. In this case, attention should also be paid to the income threshold, which requires a certain amount of income to be secured to maintain certain survival days. These findings should be considered concerning the following three points of argument.

First, most theories calling for a healthy diet and lifestyle changes were derived from previous investigations targeting adults over a wide range of ages [28, 29]. Many studies that identified significant associations between healthy lifestyles and health outcomes incorporated people in early, middle, and later adulthood [30, 31].

As a result, much evidence-based health education has also been assumed to be fully applicable to older people. Thus, we should distinguish between healthy aging led by healthy life habits during younger life periods influenced by their parents.

Second, several reports have addressed a significant association between healthy habits and health outcomes among elderly populations [32–35]. These studies focused on the relationship between healthy habits and health outcomes adjusted only for individual essential demographic variables without any attention to the confounding factors.

In comparison, our study analyzed associations between healthy habits and outcomes embedded in a model with a broader spectrum involving socioeconomic and health-related dimensional compartments resulting in control over as many potential confounds as possible for the first time until now [25, 26, 36].

Reproducibility by covariance structure analysis is expected by utilizing the results of three surveys of the same person every three years and data that clarify the survival and degree of care required after three years.

Our findings suggest, therefore, that the described associations between healthy habits and elderly healthy survival (showed **Figure 3**) might be confounded with socioeconomic status and health-related dimensional factors.

Third, although chronological analysis can reveal causal relationships among different latent variables, up until now, there have been few studies using this analysis in the gerontology research area. The current studies were the first trial to investigate causal associations by the SEM method using longitudinal data following the same subjects across six years, including survival days [25, 26, 36].

According to the standardized effects, we have been shown that dietary health and lifestyle habits did not cause healthy longevity. Longevity without bedridden status was the effect of physical, mental, and social health supported by socioeconomic status rather than a healthy diet and lifestyle (**Figure 4**).

Our study verified a solid causal association from three years earlier of three health-related dimensions toward the degree of nursing care and survival rate. Other studies have presented the expected consequence that mortality among older people is significantly associated with their physical health [19, 28], mental health [22, 35], and social health [28].

The current study incorporated the three health states into one latent variable using data from the same year (the three health-rated dimensions), as our previous reports suggest [26]. However, the reciprocal correlation among variables of the three health states does not coincidentally occur. Still, rather social health may be affected by mental health directly and by physical health indirectly in different chronological periods [36, 37].

Figure 4 shows the nearly null effect of healthy diet and lifestyle habits on healthy longevity. This finding opposed previous studies [6–12], as discussed above. However, these results are supported by the study of Diehr et al. [32] in those older adults aged 65 years and over who were overweight or obese had no worse and sometimes better outcomes in categories such as the activity of daily living, years of healthy life and active life expectancy compared to individuals of average weight.

From our perspective, it is assumed that overweight or obese conditions resulting from dietary health and lifestyle habits may have little influence on elderly health and living conditions.

Using covariance structure analysis, we analyzed the relationship between educational attainment, annual marital income, and health, namely physical, mental, and social health. As a result, it is clarified that educational attainment about half a century ago determined the annual income of married couples and that socioeconomic factors have a more decisive influence on both mental health and social health, subsequently support physical health, and ultimately affect social health.

The standardized estimate, which indicates the direct effect of socioeconomic factors on physical health, was tiny at 0.04. Forty-three percentage of social health could be explained. Analyses by gender showed almost similar results (**Figure 5**).

This new evidence would be completely new knowledge from an international perspective, and reproducibility is required.

Our research shows that the effects of educational attainment and income on healthy longevity are not direct but may have indirect effects through the three health factors (**Figure 4**). Several studies support our work. Based on the multivariate analysis, an extensive census data analysis of Estonia showed that educational differences in mortality were observed between men and women. Specifically, we showed that people with a more extended education period than those with the lowest education level were more likely to live 13.1 years longer for men and 8.6 years longer for women [38].

Manox et al. clarified through covariance variance structure analysis that educational attainment does not directly affect health but leads to health maintenance as a more indirect and distal end effect of entering a desirable occupation and maintaining income [39].

Similarly, Wardle et al. [40] reported that indexed status by occupational social class was significantly associated with favorable attitudes underlying various health behaviors and their health-sustaining effects, regardless of age or gender.

Our study shows that socioeconomic status may increase awareness, and the three desirable health factors may favor eating and lifestyle habits. In other words, favorable eating habits and lifestyle habits may not ultimately determine healthy longevity.

Instead, it was shown that economically sound groups that can maintain good eating habits and lifestyles based on desirable socioeconomic factors, especially those with sensual mental health, may be linked to healthy longevity, which is the final effect. Thus, as Manox et al. [39] pointed out, the achievement of higher education supported that it could have a distal impact on health outcomes through the expansion of social status, the type of occupation, and the potential for increased income.

This study had some limitations. In September 2001, the initial response rate was as high as 80.2%, but in the second round in September 2004, it fell to 52.0%. In particular, older people may have been missing more due to increased institutional admissions and deaths in hospitals and long-term care homes. This increase in the exclusion ratio of the target population could lead to random error and selection bias. Therefore, since excluding data with missing values would improve the fit of the model using SEM, the final analysis excluded data with one or more missing observed variables.

However, the exclusion of missing data did not change the study results. Therefore, the selection bias was insignificant even in this study, which shows missing values. It is unclear which of the three health factors indicated by the WHO has a more substantial impact on healthy longevity. As shown in **Figure 6**, socioeconomic factors can primarily strongly affect mental health and social health. However, it is entirely unclear which physical, mental, and social health factors contribute the most to healthy life expectancy. These hypotheses are our following research topics. More detailed follow-up is needed.

A review of our research yielded the following conclusions: It was revealed that healthy older people in the physical, mental, and social spheres were more likely to practice healthy eating habits and lifestyle habits. On the other hand, it was shown that a healthy diet and lifestyle might not directly affect healthy longevity, which is not required for long-term care but has a long survival day. Instead, healthy longevity could be directly affected by the three favorable health factors indicated by the WHO, which are socioeconomically supported. However, to make promising eating habits and lifestyle habits, it is necessary to maintain the three health factors supported by socioeconomic factors. Therefore, it is required to pay attention to the three health factors supported by economic independence and a healthy lifestyle strongly influenced by the three health factors.

It should be noted that socioeconomic factors are the essential foundation for the elderly to maintain healthy longevity, even if the continuation of undesirable lifestyle habits hinders healthy longevity.

As a result, attention should not be paid to the individual's only responsibility. Much more attention should be paid to public commitment to creating a supportive environment.

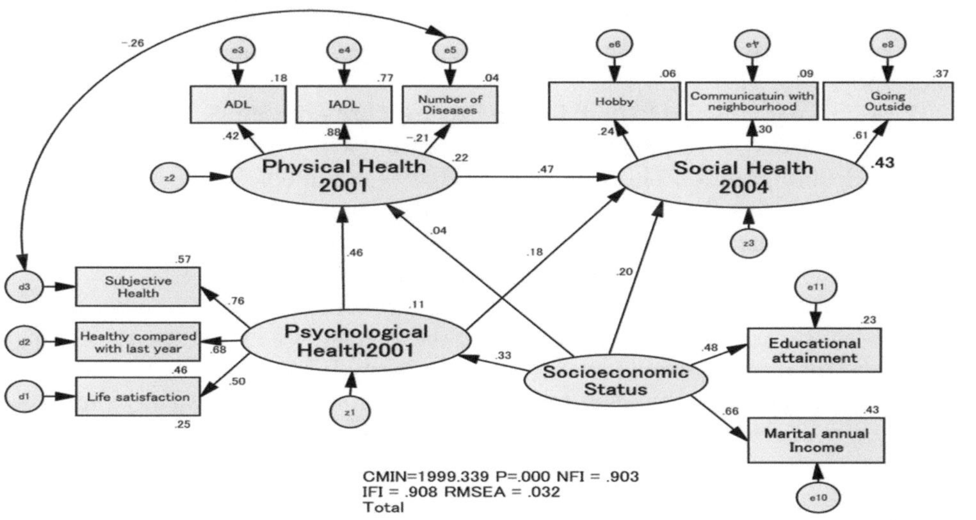

Figure 6.
Social health is a causal structure based on socioeconomic factors to support mental health and is determined through subsequent physical health for both sexes.

4.2 Marital annual income threshold to maintain survival

One of the leading scientific findings revealed by this study is that the marital yearly income threshold required to keep the number of survival days has been clarified.

In addition to showing a statistically significant relationship between income and survival days, we clarified that there is a threshold for income to maintain a certain number of survival days. For the elderly, it wa s4.5 million yen(0.0346 million US $) for both sexes as a marital yearly income.

In future research, it will be necessary to conduct an analysis based on equivalent income that considers family members, as some people live alone without a spouse. In addition, this survey did not implement survey items such as living conditions. These are a topic for future research.

Other than our previous study [25], no further research has been reported in Japan that has tracked survival concerning the amount of annual income that determines the number of survival days of individual life. Therefore, to improve the validity, additional tests are required, and reproducibility is required.

According to the 2021 Wage Structure Basic Statistical Survey [27, 41], Japan's Ministry of Health, Labor and Welfare reported the average monthly income for full-time workers in 2021 was 0.037 million Japanese yen. Twenty years ago, in 2001, the average monthly salary was 0.036 million yen. In this way, changes in the amount of personal income in Japan over time have remained almost constant over the past 20 years, making it one of the countries with a minor increase in revenue among the advanced G7 countries.

Although the increase in average life expectancy in Japan slowed down, it continued to increase to the same level as in developed countries where personal income is rising. This suggests that income alone cannot explain the factors determining extending life expectancy. This fact can also reveal that Okinawa Prefecture, which has the lowest income in Japan, had the longest average life expectancy and that Tokyo, which has the highest income city, does not have the longest average life expectancy.

The authors [42] have clarified that the average life expectancy of municipalities with a large population in Japan increases significantly with the elevation of latitude in the municipality location. This fact suggests that even if medical care in high-altitude provincial cities is not better than in urban areas, unpolluted water sources are secured, and the natural environment surrounded by abundant greenery contributes to the extension of the lifespan of living organisms.

Therefore, it is presumed that the community's natural environment and social networks are favorable factors for extending the average life expectancy, assuming that a constant income is secured and relative poverty is low.

It has been reported that other factors that determine the survival day and heredity are reflected in survival in old age about half a century later. For example, it explains the causal relationship that growth is retarded and short stature increases the mortality rate in the period when the height increases [43]. Regarding the mechanism, Davey et al. [44] reported that the socioeconomic factors of the parents in childhood reflected the nutritional status of the family, and the child's significant organs reached a level where they could fully demonstrate their functions.

Hasegawa et al. [45] reported the causal relationship between socioeconomic factors and lifestyle habits on the survival rate of urban older adults, following the survival of 8,285 people for three years. Socioeconomic factors indirectly affect healthy life maintenance via the three health factors and report the possibility that socioeconomic status is the basis of survival.

The results of this research followed previous research [12, 17, 40] that it is necessary to secure a certain level of income to maintain survival days. In the future, it will be required to verify the effects of social security policy interventions to correct health disparities.

Our studies suggest that there may be a threshold for the number of years alive and related annual income. However, the research method had limitations. In addition, many issues can be pointed out to improve the research results' validity.

As for the annual income question, objective information such as equivalent income and whole-life income should be added to consider equivalent disposable income. In addition, The next research topic is to add survey items such as subjective questions such as economic living conditions and satisfaction with health [46], which are reported to be related to survival.

A future research subject is to increase the results' internal and external validity by random sampling.

Acknowledgements

This research was supported by the Ministry of Health, Labour and Welfare (Hone0-Health-042) and the Ministry of Education, Culture, Sports, Science and Technology's Grants-in-Aid for Scientific Research (B) (Nos. 1531012 &14350327). We are also grateful for the research financial support from the Mitsubishi Foundation (2009-2021) in 2009. The author expresses special gratitude to all those who participated in the collaborative research survey between Tama City, Tokyo, and Tokyo Metropolitan University.

Conflict of interest

There is no conflict of interest status to be disclosed in this study.

Author details

Tanji Hoshi
Tokyo Metropolitan University, Tokyo, Japan

*Address all correspondence to: star@onyx.dti.ne.jp

References

[1] Mathers CD, Murray CJ, Salomon JA, Sadana R, Tandon A, Lopez AD, et al. Healthy life expectancy: Comparison of OECD countries in 2001. Australian and New Zealand Journal of Public Health. 2003;**27**:5-11

[2] Marmot MG, Smith GD. Why are the Japanese living longer? BMJ. 1989;**299**: 1547-1551

[3] Overview of the 2018 Ministry of Health, Labor and Welfare Abridged Life Tables. https://www.mhlw.go.jp/toukei/saikin/hw/life/life18/index.html (Review: 25 February 2022)

[4] Asiskovitch S. Gender and health outcomes: The impact of healthcare systems and their financing on life expectancies of women and men. Social Science & Medicine. 2010;**70**:886-895

[5] Kondo N, Mizutani T, Minai J, Kazama M, et al. Factors explaining disability-free life expectancy in Japan: The proportion of older workers, self-reported health status, and the number of public health nurses. Journal of Epidemiology. 2005;**15**:219-227

[6] A new perspective on the health of Canadians; A working document. Available from: http://www.phac-aspc.gc.ca/ph-sp/pdf/perspect-eng.pdf

[7] Healthy People; The surgeon general's report on health promotion and disease prevention. Available from: http://profiles.nlm.nih.gov/ps/access/NNBBGK.pdf

[8] Bronnum-Hansen H, Juel K, Davidsen M, Sorensen J. Impact of selected risk factors on quality-adjusted life expectancy in Denmark. Scandinavian Journal of Public Health. 2007;**35**:510-515

[9] Willcox BJ, He Q, Chen R, Yano K, Masaki KH, Grove JS, et al. Midlife risk factors and healthy survival in men. Journal of the American Medical Association. 2006;**296**:2343-2350

[10] Enstrom JE, Breslow L. Lifestyle and reduced mortality among active California Mormons, 1980-2004. Preventive Medicine. 2008;**46**:133-136

[11] Nothlings U, Ford ES, Kroger J, Boeing H. Lifestyle factors and mortality among adults with diabetes: Findings from the European prospective investigation into Cancer and nutrition-Potsdam study. Journal of Diabetes. 2010;**2**:112-117

[12] Tamakoshi A, Kawado M, Ozasa K, Tamakoshi K, Lin Y, Yagyu K, et al. Impact of smoking and other lifestyle factors on life expectancy among japanese: Findings from the Japan collaborative cohort (JACC) study. Journal of Epidemiology. 2010;**20**: 370-376

[13] Hoi le V, Phuc HD, Dung TV, Chuc NT, Lindholm L. Remaining life expectancy among older people in a rural area of Vietnam: Trends and socioeconomic inequalities during a period of multiple transitions. BMC Public Health. 2009;**9**:471

[14] Matthews RJ, Jagger C, Hancock RM. Does socio-economic advantage lead to a longer, healthier old age? Social Science & Medicine. 2006;**62**:2489-2499

[15] Jagger C, Gillies C, Moscone F, Cambois E, Van Oyen H, Nusselder W, et al. Inequalities in healthy life years in the 25 countries of the European Union in 2005: A cross-national meta-regression analysis. Lancet. 2008;**372**: 2124-2131

[16] Sugiura Y, Ju YS, Yasuoka J, Jimba M. Rapid increase in Japanese life expectancy after world war II. Bioscience Trends. 2010;**4**:9-16

[17] Kagamimori S, Gaina A, Nasermoaddeli A. Socioeconomic status and health in the Japanese population. Social Science & Medicine. 2009;**68**: 2152-2160

[18] International Health Conference: The Constitution of the World Health Organization. New York; 1946

[19] Byberg L, Melhus H, Gedeborg R, Sundstrom J, et al. Total mortality after changes in leisure time physical activity in 50 year old men: 35 year follow-up of population based cohort. British Journal of Sports Medicine. 2009;**43**:482

[20] Donaldson LJ, Jagger C. Survival and functional capacity: Three year follow up of an elderly population in hospitals and homes. Journal of Epidemiology and Community Health. 1983;**37**:176-179

[21] Eplov LF, Jorgensen T, Birket-Smith M, Segel S, et al. Mental vulnerability as a predictor of early mortality. Epidemiology. 2005;**16**:226-232

[22] Kaplan GA, Goldberg DE, Everson SA, Cohen RD, et al. Perceived health status and morbidity and mortality: Evidence from the Kuopio ischaemic heart disease risk factor study. International Journal of Epidemiology. 1996;**25**:259-265

[23] Khaw KT, Wareham N, Bingham S, Welch A, et al. Combined impact of health behaviours and mortality in men and women: The EPIC-Norfolk prospective population study. PLoS Medicine. 2008;**5**:12

[24] Seeman TE, Kaplan GA, Knudsen L, Cohen R, Guralnik J. Social network ties and mortality among the elderly in the Alameda County study. American Journal of Epidemiology. 1987;**126**: 714-723

[25] Hoshi T, Kodama S, Kurimori S, Fujita K. Married annual income threshold for survival days among. Both elderly suburban and rural dwellers. Fortune Journal of Health Sciences. 2022; **5**(3):529-541

[26] Hoshi T. SES. Dietary and lifestyle habits, three health-related dimensions, and healthy survival days. In: Hoshi T, Kodama S, editors. The Structure of Healthy Life Determinants: Lessons from the Japanese Aging Cohort Studies. Singapore: Springer; 2018. pp. 134-189

[27] World development report 2006. Equity and Development. The World Bank Oxdord University Press. World Bank Group Open Knowledge Repository. Available from: https://openknowledge.worldbank.org/handle/10986/5988 [Review: 11 July 2022]

[28] Berkman LF, Breslow L. Health and Ways on Living; the Alameda County Study. New York: Oxford University Press; 1983

[29] Ford ES, Zhao G, Tsai J, Li C. Low-risk lifestyle Behaviors and all-cause mortality: Findings from the National Health and nutrition examination survey III mortality study. American Journal of Public Health. 2011;**101**(10):1922-1929. DOI: 10.2105/AJPH.2011.300167

[30] Millen BE, Quatromoni PA, Pencina M, Kimokoti R, et al. Unique dietary patterns and chronic disease risk profiles of adult men: The Framingham nutrition studies. Journal of the American Dietetic Association. 2005;**105**:1723-1734

[31] Dam RM, Li T, Spiegelman D, Franco OH, et al. Combined impact of lifestyle factors on mortality: Prospective

cohort study in US women. BMJ. 2008; **337**:a1440

[32] Diehr P, O'Meara ES, Fitzpatrick A, Newman AB, et al. Weight, mortality, years of healthy life, and active life expectancy in older adults. Journal of the American Geriatrics Society. 2008;**56**: 76-83

[33] Iestra J, Knoops K, Kromhout D, de Groot L, et al. Lifestyle, Mediterranean diet and survival in European post-myocardial infarction patients. European Journal of Cardiovascular Prevention and Rehabilitation. 2006;**13**:894-900

[34] Knoops KT, de Groot LC, Kromhout D, Perrin AE, et al. Mediterranean diet, lifestyle factors, and 10-year mortality in elderly European men and women: The HALE project. Journal of the American Medical Association. 2004;**292**:1433-1439

[35] Spiers N, Jagger C, Clarke M, Arthur A. Are gender differences in the relationship between self-rated health and mortality enduring? Results from three birth cohorts in Melton Mowbray, United Kingdom. The Gerontologist. 2003;**43**:406-411 discussion 372-405

[36] Hoshi T, Ryu S, Fujiwara Y. Urban health and determinant factors for longer life for the elderly urban dwellers in Tokyo. In: Proceedings of the International Symposium on Sustainable Urban Environment. Tokiyo: Metropolitan University; 2007. pp. 61-66

[37] Hoshi T, Takagi C, Bosako Y, Nakayama N, et al. Chronological evaluation of physical, psychological and social health of urban elderly dwellers over 6 years and assesment of cuasal inter-relationships. Nihon Koshu Eisei Zasshi. 2011;**58**:491-500

[38] Leinsalu M, Vagero D, Kunst AE. Estonia 1989-2000: Enormous increase in mortality differences by education. International Journal of Epidemiology. 2003;**32**:1081-1087

[39] Singh-Manoux A, Clarke P, Marmot M. Multiple measures of socio-economic position and psychosocial health: Proximal and distal measures. International Journal of Epidemiology. 2002;**31**:1192-1199 discussion 1199-1200

[40] Wardle J, Steptoe A. Socioeconomic differences in attitudes and beliefs about healthy lifestyles. Journal of Epidemiology and Community Health. 2003;**57**:440-443

[41] 2021 Wage Structure Basic Statistics Survey Ministry of Health, Labor and Welfare. Available from: https://news.yahoo.co.jp/articles/226d8885b45364a7c4b0399e522182c6a82f2a28

[42] Hoshi T, Taniguchi R. A study on the relationship between average life expectancy and altitude in municipalities nationwide. Proceedings of the Annual Meeting of the Japanese Society of Public Health. 2003;**62**:183

[43] Flegal KM, Graubard BI, Williamson DF, et al. Excess deaths associated with underweight, overweight, and obesity. JAMA. 2005; **293**:1861-1867

[44] Davey Smith G, Hart C, Upton M, Hole D. Height and risk of death among men and women: Aetiological implications of associations with cardiorespiratory disease and cancer mortality. Journal of Epidemiology and Community Health. 2000;**54**:97-113

[45] Hasegawa T, Takashi T, Hoshi T, et al. The effects of socioeconomic status and lifestyle on life expectancy: A structural analysis of an elderly Japanese population. International Medical Journal. 2011;**18**(4):261-264

[46] Montano D. Socioeconomic status, well-being and mortality: A comprehensive life course analysis of panel data, Germany, 1984-2016.Arch. Public Health. 2021;**79**(1):40. DOI: 10.1186/s13690-021-00559-7

Chapter 5

A Salutogenic Approach for Collaboration in Health and Technology

Arild Berg, Safora Johansen, Anne Lund, Michael Alexander Riegler and Jorunn Marie Andersen

Abstract

Through collaboration, health services and health-promoting environments can be influenced by patients, health professionals, and stakeholders. Antonovsky's concept of salutogenesis includes the promotion of a sense of coherence, where the feeling of meaningfulness and people's ability to influence their own situation is central. These concepts were the units of analysis in this embedded case study, including an educational project analyzed in relation to relevant research projects. The educational project was the development of a new master course, "Interaction in health and technology," for students with different background in health-related education, including radiography, occupational therapy, biomedicine, biomedical laboratory science, artificial intelligence, and design. Through a qualitative content analysis, pitfalls and success criteria for collaboration in health and technology within a salutogenic theoretical framework were identified. These included user understanding of diagnostic value by artificial intelligence through visualization, user journeys for better health services, patient opinions about assistive technology, and developing understandable AI models. An interdisciplinary understanding of a sense of coherence as described in this study can strengthen collaboration in health and technology. The results of the current case study show also the potential for replication of the approach in different sites in various countries.

Keywords: occupational therapy, design, higher education, biomedicine, interdisciplinary collaboration, radiography, artificial intelligence, innovation

1. Introduction: new ways of understanding approaches to health and technologies

New technologies have affected our insight to health, including new ways of understanding approaches to health research systems [1]. The definition of health technology is according to World Health Organization (WHO) "the application of organized knowledge and skills in the form of devices, medicines, vaccines, procedures and systems developed to solve a health problem and improve quality of life." [2]. As a subcategory assistive technology is defined by WHO as "the application of organized knowledge and skills related to assistive products, including systems and services" [3]. Traditionally, in public health services, both principles and approaches have varied through time [4, 5]. From a philosophy of science perspective, both quantitative and qualitative methodological approaches have been used [6]. Participation and co-creation are needed to ensure that users, such as health professionals and patients, can take part in and influence new and improved solutions [7]. It is often an aim to develop methods in health where patients should be included in the validation of results before scaling up technology, for example, in advanced technology such as radiography [8]. From a technological perspective, there is a need for new thinking in education because new practices emerge with innovative technology [9]. An example is artificial intelligence, which is currently influencing higher education and the health sector. Critical reflections on new technologies and solutions are important to adapt to a new working life, where innovations are needed both locally and globally [10]. Due to general growth in societal complexity, the need for interdisciplinary education is growing [11] as well as knowledge about collaboration and co-creation [10]. Challenges in this matter are that professions change and therefore there is a need for critical studies about how to succeed in this matter. One way to achieve this is through a salutogenic approach, a concept introduced by Antonovsky [12]. Historically, this included the ability to use the resources available, as a sense of coherence. Today, Antonovsky's theory has influenced several societal practices, including both health and technology [13]. The use of Antonovskys theory and ontological position can be valuable in future health research as it integrates people in interaction with their environment as well as experiencing chaos and change as a normal state of life [13]. The salutogenic approach will contribute to flexible choices and possibilities for adopting to change for health professionals in a complex society.

2. Background: Changing positions between professions

Andrew Abbott developed a theory about the system of professions [14] concerning how expertise is changing in working life. He addressed how different professions have interacted through the ages and how new professions challenge previous professions as society evolves. He says that with an ecological perspective on professions, one can see professions in relation to how they grow through niches. Professions transform and leave a niche, opening up for new professions. He believes that professional history is characterized by struggles to occupy different niches. Abbott describes that there have been disciplines where certain professions have had precedence and that this has often been linked to the legal level, from which professional policymakers have asked for advice. Furthermore, he says that the professions together form a system so that they replace each other as society evolves and that the professions move, invading areas that appear to be more appropriate. Further, he describes that there are three levels in particular that this unfolds. The first level is in the workplace, the second level is in society; in the culture and general perception of society, and finally at the third level, it is in relation to laws and administrative rules [14].

There is such a change in positions between different professions, but also internally within the health systems, there are changes of professions, shown in a study about the coordination between health service professions [15]. The study demonstrates how the health service in Norway often is characterized by an increasing fragmentation of specialization, emphasizing the importance of developing interactions and relationships between people that are characterized by equality, respectful mindset, and reciprocity knowledge. The study shows how four forms of collaboration can contribute to better health services, and these four are relational collaboration, coordinated task distribution, operationally closed collaboration, and fragmented task distribution. Relational cooperation is characterized by closeness and interconnection. Operationally closed cooperation is characterized by proximity and differentiation, where you work more separately. In a coordinated distribution of tasks, there is a long distance between the parties and participants cooperate from such distance with their own distinct tasks. Finally, fragmented task distribution is also characterized by both distance and differentiation, but here there are fewer meeting places both physically and digitally and little reciprocity knowledge. The conclusion of this study is that there are two types of interactions, ranging from fragmented task distribution to relational collaboration. The study shows that is not the conflict between understandings that is the main challenge for the interaction, but the lack of such a conflict. This is supported by literature on teamwork where stages of multidisciplinary team building in public health are characterized by Forming – Storming – Norming – Performing [16], where storming includes potential situations of conflict, such as discussions. Therefore, it can be important to not avoid conflicts but to strive for negotiations and discussions that highlight differences to achieve a real mutual understanding and reciprocity competence and respect for each other's work.

2.1 Co-innovation in higher education

In higher education, there is a need to address changes in each education to adapt to a changing working life, and bring about overarching innovations [17]. An example of such innovation potential is described in a study concerning a trans-disciplinary approach for co-innovation in social science and artificial intelligence [17]. It shows how there should be greater cooperation between international industrial cooperation and transnational university cooperation in larger sustain-able ecosystems. This has synergies where, for example, machine learning and artificial intelligence can help make this synergy happen. The study refers to how the EU and China cooperation in technology and innovation has been tested. Their proposals for a transdisciplinary approach include both multiple disciplines and research fields, a transnational innovation ecosystem coupled with the civic engagement of universities. This is formed through international relations and various models of innovation where also institutional category and social network theory, social networks, analyses, and professional matching are important. Their long-term goal is to use artificial intelligence that can predict and propose potential and suitable universities and industry partners in international collaborations. This article is on a conceptual level, and the authors would like to discuss case studies with more practical examples.

2.2 The course: interaction in health and technology

Part of this objective is touched upon in this study, with a case study that includes a new university course in a new master's program in health and technology. The course name is "Interactions in health and technology." In order to achieve an inter-disciplinary approach to topics concerning health and technology, it is valuable for students to discover common ground. A patient journey could serve as a common starting point with an aim for health and the will to do something good for the patient as a common context. Additionally, a health-promoting perspective in a wide sense could be used and applied in this chapter. The course was made for students with different backgrounds in health-related education, including radiography, occupational therapy, biomedicine, biomedical laboratory science, artificial intelligence, and design. International, national health and welfare schemes were used as a starting point for the education of professionals with new interdisciplinary competence that can solve growing welfare problems, including the aging population and new user groups, in the health sector. Because new technology is constantly being used in the health sector, being able to understand the technology and being able to talk to and collaborate with different professionals in the field is important. This applies both to relationships with users and patients, but also between professionals. The rapid technological development in the health sector requires better and new types of interaction between different actors to promote better and more efficient health services.

In the course, it was therefore necessary that students learn about technological development, system design, and service innovation. Both public and private actors can contribute with experiences and cases, but also other areas are relevant, such as specialist health services, municipal health services, the business sector, and other interest organizations. Students will through different cases explore how new technology contributes to sustainable solutions in health and care services and think and reflect on ethical challenges that arise when new technology is adopted. Interdisciplinary collaboration competence in the development and implementation of new technology in health and social services was emphasized in the course. Some of the things the student should know are, for example, to explain key concepts related to technological development, system design, and service innovation. Some skills they will learn in the course are to be able to discuss and evaluate established and new relevant methods in research and creative development work in health technology, but also to be able to discuss health technology as socially responsible innovation and research, RRI [18]. An important general competence in the course was that the student can reflect on and fit their own professional background, identity, and competence in an interdisciplinary context. By being able to reflect on user perspectives and professional identity from traditional and new perspectives, the student can identify opportunities for innovation processes within their own field of study and propose new solutions, work methods, services, or product-based innovation projects. In this way, the student can contribute to a user orientation of system design through critical thinking. Further, the student should use a suitable conceptual framework that promotes interdisciplinary interaction and contributes to interdisciplinary teamwork. A qualitative content analysis of the professional fields in the course was studied from a salutogenic perspective.

2.3 A salutogenic approach

A health-promoting way of thinking was developed by Antonovsky [12], where his principle of salutogenesis is about the path to health rather than thinking about the path to disease. Antonovsky studied concentration camp survivors after World War II and asked them what made them able to create a meaningful life even after horrific experiences. He found that those who fared best had created a connectedness in their lives, a sense of coherence. This has become a well-known concept that has formed the basis for many holistic and overarching approaches in the field of health [5, 13].

A sense of coherence is including what is meaningful and understandable, and the opportunity to influence and change a situation or one's own life situation, such as an illness. The more a person is able to understand and fit in a suitable way into what they are supposed to do, the more it contributes to an increased degree of understanding. This is also about how you manage to create a meaningful whole in what you do, and how you feel or experience that the process connected to an illness is meaningful. The more individuals manage to handle a situation or their illness, it will strengthen the person's own health development and experience of being able to survive even a difficult situation.

The research question in this study is therefore how to collaborate in health technology with a salutogenic approach. The study will show some cases of what sense of coherence means in different professions, and how these different professions can collaborate.

3. Methods: embedded case study

In this case study, we want to unfold the concepts of salutogenesis related to a course that has been developed in the field of health and technology, where multidisciplinary groups are represented. This applies to physiotherapists, professionals in biomedicine, biomedical laboratory scientists, radiographers, artificial intelligence engineers, designers, and occupational therapists. These professions have traditions from both qualitative and quantitative research, so they are well suited to specifying what these concepts may mean in practice, because the examples may have transfer value to other interdisciplinary arenas for cooperation.

This case study [19] included literature studies, archival studies, artifacts, and participatory observation. We aimed for a deeper understanding of what salutogenesis can mean in interdisciplinary collaboration in health and technology through different work groups in an interdisciplinary team [20].

The scientific approach is based on a tradition in Hermeneutics or the way people understand the world and context they are situated in [21]. The philosopher Gadamer was concerned that in science as well as in everyday life, it was difficult to understand the world around you without taking with you the background you already have. You are characterized by your culture, upbringing, education, and also your field of study. Gadamer introduced the concept of preconceptions, fore meanings, which deals with our past experience as a prerequisite for our understanding, and also what he called the "horizon of understanding." Our horizon of understanding is a concept describing the limit of our understanding. He was concerned that we will never escape our own background and that we all have a limited understanding, but that it is possible to try to achieve a fusion of horizons of understanding, where one approaches in understanding each other. From a hermeneutic perspective, one can aim for a mutual understanding into a "fusion of horizons"; where in Gadamer's words the "old and new are always combining into something of living value, without either being explicitly foregrounded from the other" [21]. This view has been developed into post-phenomenology by Ihde, who recognized that people understand the world through technology, both advanced technology and less complex technology, such as glasses [22].

It is a goal to collaborate in health sciences, which increasingly collaborate with other disciplines, especially within technology. Mutual understanding and interest in other fields is a necessity. As technology becomes more and more advanced, the user-oriented approach from design professions stands for an important approach [23–25]. This user-oriented approach is also related to the individual's self-understanding, and empathy toward others understanding, as Antonovsky was concerned with, that you are part of a larger context, and that you have the opportunity to understand what you are a part of and how you can influence it. This is also a goal for people concerned with health and technology, both professionals, students, and patients.

Through such collaboration, it is conceivable that one should promote not only a pleasant and interdisciplinary tone, there are also ideas [15, 16] that want to promote the challenges and perhaps that collaborators should deliberately try to use different ways of understanding health, as a way to increase understanding of each other's differences and horizons of understanding, in line with Gadamer's ideas. In these studies [15, 16], conflict in group processes can be seen as a learning process that can strengthen interdisciplinary cooperation in the long term. To aim for, and to tolerate, seeing different points of view, creates a pedagogical challenge where students and professionals must both promote their own field of study, but also try to find a place in an interaction between different professionals, in a professional life that is constantly changing.

Through the study, we will identify different variations of sense of coherence, influence, and meaningfulness through an embedded case study with pattern matching [19]. The theoretical framework consists of subunits of analysis, the key components, connecting both success criteria with critical success factors as described in the Project Excellence Model [26]. The key components in this study have been connecting Antonovskys concepts, with pedagogical approaches. This included combining a sense of coherence, meaningfulness, and ability to influence a situation, with pedagogical approaches of Forming – Storming – Norming – Performing [16]. This was further discussed into problem-based learning, because this was suitable in such a dynamic context based on real problems in professional and working life, including diagnostic, treatment, and training, as well as health promotion both in the health care setting and in the community, where unique solutions must be developed every time [27].

3.1 Findings: exploring a sense of coherence through a multidisciplinary lens

We used articles and studies that are relevant to the case we have chosen: the topic sense of coherence in an interdisciplinary interaction course in health and technology touching upon user experience, diagnostics, treatment, healthcare services, communities, and research. In this study, we present articles that deal with interdisciplinarity and thus elaborate on the concept of sense of coherence from some selected areas; radiation therapy, physiotherapy, artificial intelligence, design, biomedicine, biomedical laboratory science, and occupational therapy. The purpose of this study is to show some examples from some chosen areas of professional expertise. This has an essential value for the chosen areas. Although they are specific, they represent a broad range of disciplines and demonstrate the variation of the fore understanding [21] of the same concept.

In the study, we thus see different examples of what a sense of coherence means in different disciplines in interaction in health technology, and we place special emphasis on a sense of coherence, meaningfulness, and people's ability to influence sustainable development.

3.2 A radiography perspective

The first example we will refer to is from diagnostics where phantoms (**Figure 1**) and computer tomography (CT) technology are used [8]. CT is an X-ray machine using ionizing radiation for imaging. Ionizing radiation can be harmful to humans and should be held as low as possible. It is therefore not possible to test the impact of different CT parameters on image quality and patient dose by scanning patients in an experimental setting. Therefore, anthropomorphic phantoms are used by professionals and students to perform experimental scans in order to optimize the CT protocols used in routine CT examination of different human body parts. In this way, we avoid exposing human body parts to unnecessary radiation doses, which can be harmful and result in late side effects, such as radiation-induced cancer. The phantom used by an interdisciplinary group consisting of radiologists, physicists, radiographers, and students involved in the experiment will contribute to a close collaboration and understanding of a common goal, which in this case is to improve CT protocol optimization and improvement of patient treatment as a result of it. The phantom will also contribute to build up a feeling of mastering and coping, as well as establishment of an interaction between the team members. In other words, the phantom can be seen as an example of an interdisciplinary artifact (**Figure 2**), a boundary object [28] where different professionals can connect to understand a phenomenon with different backgrounds. Another example is using digital questionnaires, which can also be interdisciplinary where one looks at how one can use a digital tool to gain a deeper understanding of a topic. In this example, a questionnaire was used to explore the psychological impacts of COVID-19 on radiation technologists in Norway and Canada [29]. Boundary objects in this context can be an object such as a phantom or a method such as a digital questionnaire.

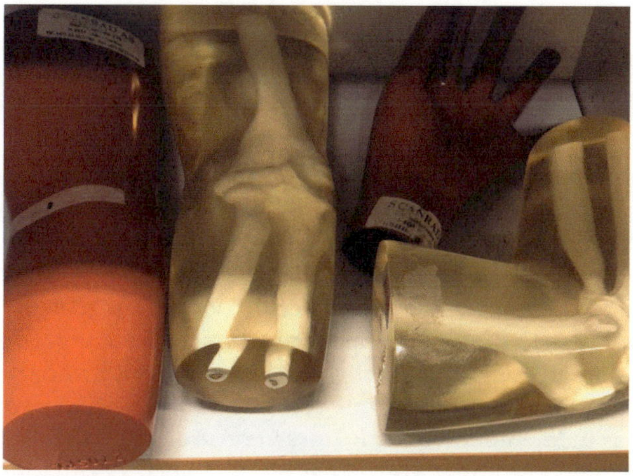

Figure 1.
Phantoms, detail.

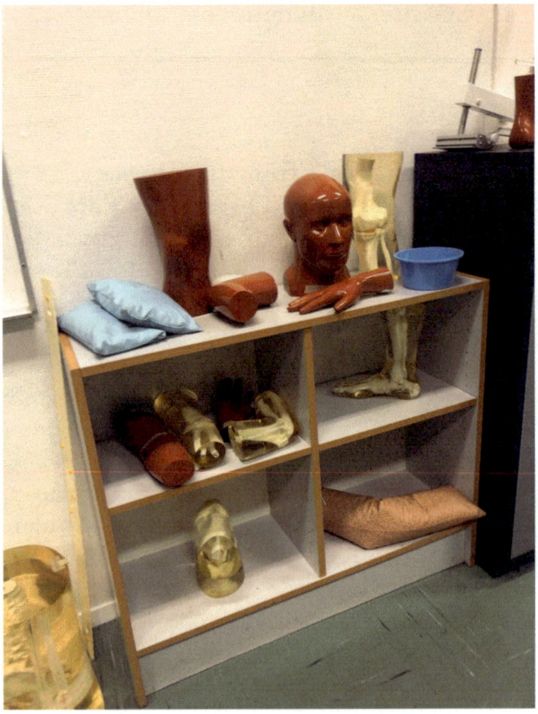

Figure 2.
Phantom collection.

3.3 An occupational therapy perspective

Other examples of using this salutogenic approach are related to health promotion, both in healthcare settings and in communities. In occupational therapy, humans are seen as active beings, taking part in, and creating, meaningful activities resulting in improved health, quality of life, and well-being [30]. This can be seen as another way of understanding the sense of coherence raised by Antonovsky. The process of implementing technologies in people's lives is very complex and elaborates on interactions between actors in the field. In occupational therapy, studies have also been conducted by working user oriented and involving older adults in technology research and development. We present two examples where qualitative methods are applied.

Example 1 elaborates on that digital assistive technology has the potential to support older adults who depend upon community healthcare services. In the Assisted Living Project, we engaged older adults in co-creating knowledge about users' needs to guide the development of technological solutions [31]. In this study, user engagement was applied and aligns with the term occupational engagement [30] meaning to involve oneself or participate in occupations to create meaning. User engagement is an important strategy toward facilitating dialog, reflexivity, and the co-creation of knowledge, it can cast users in separate roles: as informants, as partners with researchers, and as independent investigators in relation to researchers as mentors [32]. To ensure the co-creation of knowledge about diverse occupations over a 3-year period, as well as considering older adults as experts on their own lives, we considered user engagement as a partnership arguing that co-creation entails engaging citizens in actively taking part in innovation processes aimed at creating new and improved solutions for society [7]. The project demonstrates that older adults with impairments could meaningfully contribute with opinions on their needs. Applying a critical occupational perspective raised awareness regarding sociocultural assumptions about older adults in assisted living as frail and unable to participate, which may reinforce ageist and ableist stereotypes, as well as promote occupational injustice. This can also be related to that the participants created a sense of coherence and meaningfulness related to Antonovsky.

Example 2 is about involving older adults in technology research and development discussions through dialog cafés [33]. Citizen involvement is important for ensuring the relevance and quality of many research and innovation efforts. Literature shows that inadequate citizen involvement poses an obstacle during the research, development, and implementation of assistive technology. Previous studies have addressed the advantages and disadvantages of citizen engagement in health research and technology development, and there is concern about how to ensure valuable engagement to avoid situations where they do not have influence. Older adults are often excluded from being active partners in research projects. The overall objective of this project is to describe a case where dialog cafés were used as a method for involving assisted living residents in technology discussions, with the following research question: In what ways are dialog cafés useful for directing research and development and for engaging residents in assisted living facilities in assistive technology discussions? Six dialog cafés with assisted living residents (aged between 65 and 92) as participants were carried out over a period of 3 years (2016–2019). Reports that were written after each café by the group leaders and rapporteurs provide the material for the analyses in this paper.

This study demonstrates an example of facilitating user involvement where the participants felt useful by contributing to research and discussions on assistive technology and where this contribution in fact directed the research and development of the overall Assisted Living Project. This study also shows.

that dialog cafés enable older residents at an assisted living facility to contribute with opinions about their needs and perspectives on assistive technologies. This negates the view of older adults as too frail to participate and demonstrates the importance of including and collaborating with older adults in research. The findings can also be related to the fact that the participants created a sense of coherence and meaning by participating in the dialog cafés in line with the salutogenetic perspective by Antonovsky.

3.4 A perspective of artificial intelligence and biomedicine

A sense of coherence perspective can be applied to interdisciplinary work within biomedicine and artificial intelligence (AI), including the process of creating a collective understanding of the task at hand and interpreting the data resulting from the AI algorithms in a biological and patient-related context. The integration of AI in healthcare has the potential to revolutionize diagnostics, treatment, and patient care both in hospitals and in-home services for patients. However, interdisciplinary collaboration between medical professionals and AI experts is essential for the successful implementation of such technologies. The following examples show some challenges, highlighting the importance of interdisciplinary collaboration and suggesting potential pedagogical approaches.

The first example is using machine learning for predicting exposure to tacrolimus, an immunosuppressive drug, for individual dose adaptations in kidney-transplanted patients [34]. In this study, machine learning techniques are employed to estimate tacrolimus exposure in kidney transplant recipients. The success of this approach relies on the collaboration between AI experts who design the algorithms and healthcare professionals who understand the clinical context and the pharmacokinetics of the drug. The challenges in the project were that different terminologies and methodologies used by AI experts and healthcare professionals may lead to misunderstandings. In an educational setting, balancing the technical aspects of AI and the clinical aspects of healthcare can be difficult.

The second example was a project about human reproduction, including embryo and sperm motility assessment using AI algorithms. Semen analysis is used as a part of male infertility assessment and the analysis protocols are standardized by the World Health Organization (WHO) [35]. This study used deep convolutional neural networks to predict sperm motility categories based on videos captured with a microscope-mounted camera [36]. Motility assessment of sperm is an important parameter in infertility investigations and the collaboration between AI experts and medical professionals was crucial in designing and evaluating the performance of these networks. For the AI-experts, it was important to understand some biological concepts and observe the samples together with the medical experts. This could be done using a discussion microscope (**Figure 3**) or looking at video clips. Another aspect is to investigate which part of the video was used by the AI model to ensure that a meaningful part of the image is analyzed by AI (**Figure 4**). This also leads potentially to a more visual understanding of what the algorithms actually are producing compared to showing numbers of difficult to interpret metrics.

Challenges in this project included the need for extensive training of the AI models to ensure accurate and reproducible results in both AI and a biological context. Furthermore, ensuring that AI models align with the standards and guidelines set in the WHO protocols. Relevant approaches for educational purposes would be integrating AI and biomedical concepts in the curriculum to expose students to the interdisciplinary nature of the field, utilizing case studies, simulations (**Figure 4**), or collaborative projects, to provide students with hands-on experience in interdisciplinary problem-solving.

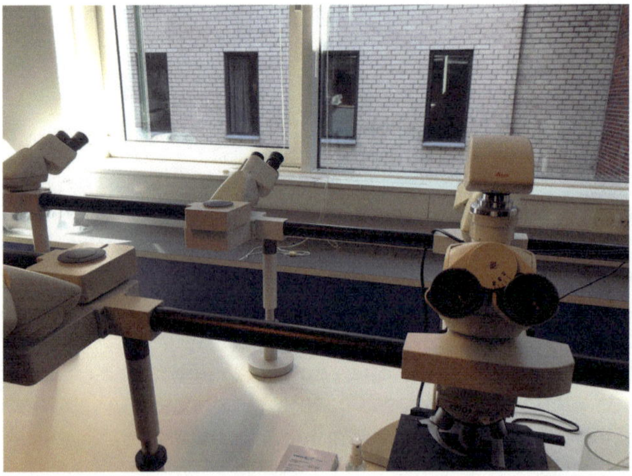

Figure 3.
Discussion microscope.

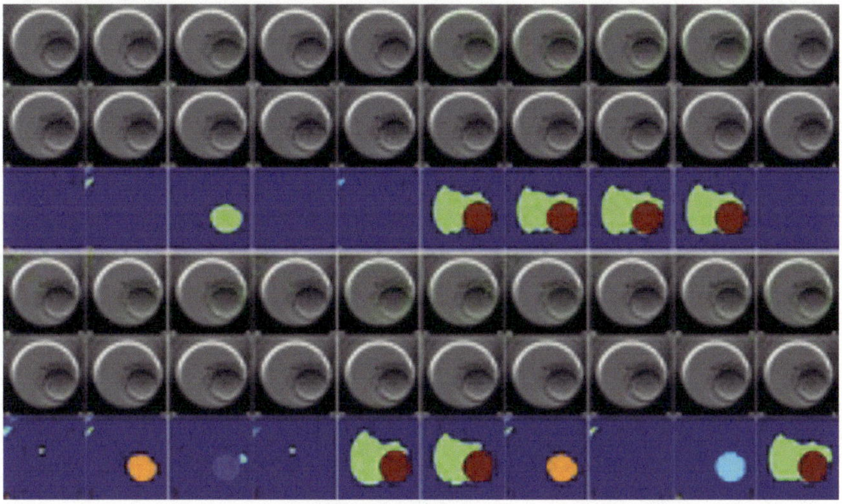

Figure 4.
Visualization of output from image analysis by an AI algorithm.

Interdisciplinary research and teaching in the context of AI, biomedicine and healthcare can be challenging due to differences in terminology, methodologies, and educational backgrounds. In addition, there is also a dramatic difference in the ethical aspects of different disciplines. Medical sciences have a culture of ethical behavior and commitment to the patient's best outcome, whereas in technology this is radically less developed. With the fact that algorithms become a part of our daily life, technologists also need to understand and develop a culture of ethical considerations focused on implications of the products they built. However, pedagogical approaches like Problem-Based Learning (PBL) [27] and the Forming-Storming-Norming-Performing stages of team building [16], can help students navigate these challenges and develop the interdisciplinary skills necessary for successful collaboration and a better cross-disciplinary understanding. By fostering a salutogenic approach, educators can promote a sense of coherence, and a deeper understanding in their students, empowering them to create innovative solutions in the ever-evolving fields of AI and healthcare.

3.5 A design perspective

An example of a user-oriented approach is the PACER research project on patient-centered engineering in rehabilitation. Here, four PhD students collaborated; a physiotherapist, an artificial intelligence engineer, a designer, and a medical technology engineer, studying what it takes to achieve good interaction between them [37]. Functional near-infrared spectroscopy (fNIRS) was designed as a cap where patients can wear to measure brain activity (**Figure 5**). Tests were done in a motion analysis laboratory (**Figure 6**). Technology and user experience were often not connected, and the aim of the project included new educational perspectives and participatory design related to patients' everyday activities. Some of the studies emphasized comprehensiveness and coherence, but other studies were more related to a monodisciplinary professional expertise that in many ways did not include the same understanding of coherence and context. For example, it was not always

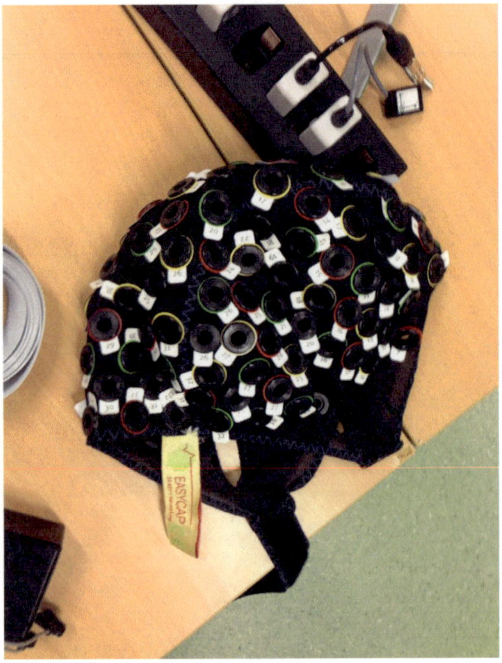

Figure 5.
Cap for fNIRS.

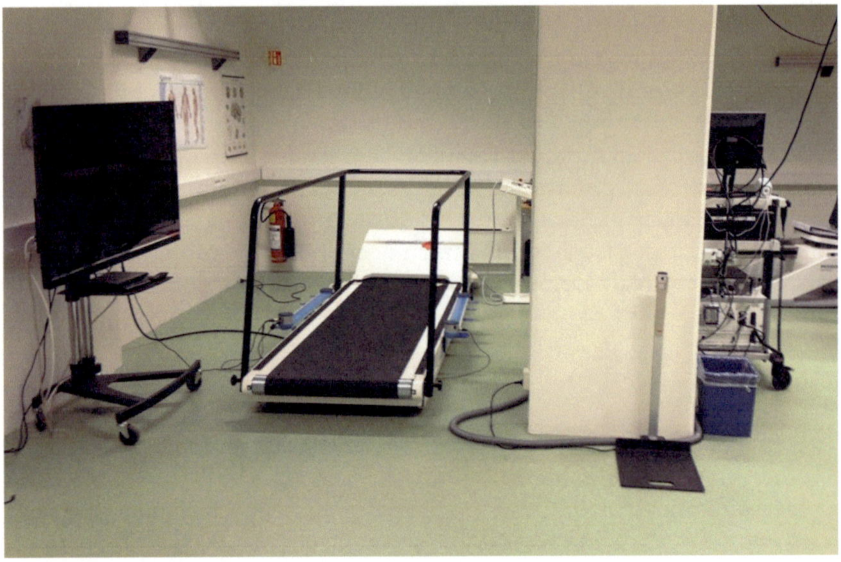

Figure 6.
Motion analysis laboratory.

relevant for someone who is developing logarithms in artificial intelligence to have a clear understanding of how the logarithms should be used in relation to a patient [38]. Nevertheless, this can be an appropriate way to put people together because they learn about different scientific traditions, different criteria for research, and different basic principles and approaches in health, where understanding the world through technology is relevant as a postphenomenological perspective [22].

In the same way as testing a product in relation to a user [37], it is also possible to test a user-oriented approach of a patient in health services. For example, service design is an approach that is often used in the development of services by a commercial product. It can be how a customer experiences ordering a product, using the product, getting it repaired, and being able to return it for recycling. In the same way, a patient in relation to a health service can also be seen as a person who should experience both acknowledging their own illness, contacting the hospital, being led through a system, and receiving the right treatment. In all these stages, there are meetings between people, meetings between people and technology, and meetings between different professionals, where there is the possibility of improving the service or improving the product. The user experience is connected to the "front stage" activities, but the premises for the treatment often happen in the "back stage" activities, including technology and diagnosis processes. People often have a deep knowledge of their own situation and needs, which is why a user-oriented approach to service design has become increasingly common in health services [37, 38].

4. Discussion: success criteria and educational perspectives

In the discussion, we will look at different success criteria [26] for interdisciplinary collaboration in health and technology. In the model shown earlier, conflict can be a step on the way in the process of understanding each other. Possible conflicts in the examples we have shown are different understandings of what constitutes comprehensiveness and coherence, what are the responsibilities and roles of the various professionals in a larger context, and how they should influence their own situation and the situation of others in the process. In other words, it is not the case that the participants in the health and technology field should only accept the technologies that exist in the world today, but one should try to have critical reflections on how one can renew and improve both technology and ways of doing things, both the technological competence in interaction with the relational competence. Guiding process concepts in the pattern matching analysis [19] related to success criteria were salutogenic concepts related to Forming, Storming, Norming, and Performing (**Table 1**).

The identified concepts were related to the success criteria of project implementation [26], such as Forming, Storming, Norming, and Performing [16].

Forming the group should be related to formal requirements for health, environment, and security. Further, everyday activities can be a starting point using qualitative approaches to understand patient situations and promote health. In interdisciplinary collaboration, the participants understanding of diagnostic value can be strengthened through visualization and communication. A topic should be seen from various interdisciplinary perspectives. The group should understand the need for interdisciplinary collaboration.

In the storming, part possible divergent views should be enhanced, and these might be related to formalized procedures. Patient opinions about assistive technology can also lead to discussion. At this stage, the aim is to strengthen dialog and reflexivity to avoid misunderstandings.

In the norming stage, an aim is to have matured about the topic and process, and to learn about each other's areas. This requires an awareness regarding participants' own sociocultural assumptions [13]. Both dialog and reflexivity should be used for

Salutogenic concepts	Concepts for collaboration	Examples from cases
Sense of coherence	Collaboration with medical equipment	Phantom used by a interdisciplinary group
	Boundary objects	Digital questionnaire, phantoms
	Visual technology for common understanding,	Discussion microscope, images, and videos
	User understanding of diagnostic value by artificial intelligence through visualization	Visualizing the part of an image used by an AI algorithm
	Using advanced visualization technology for diagnosis	Computer Tomography (CT) technology for X-ray imaging
	Service design and user journey	Back-stage activities and front-stage activities, patient experiences in a rehabilitation process
	Globalization in health research and education	Collaboration between Canadian and Norwegian researchers
Meaning-fulness	Health, environment, and security	Using phantoms to minimize radiation exposure
	Contribution to improve diagnostics and patient treatment	Using AI for diagnostics
	Everyday activities and qualitative approaches to promote health	Taking part in and creating meaningful activities
	Deliver community health care services in line with users' needs through dialog and reflexivity	Dialog cafes with users
	Patient opinions about assistive technology	User experience with assistive technology
	awareness regarding sociocultural assumptions	Dialog cafes for engaging elderly people in technology development
	Treatment based on interdisciplinary collaboration	Predicting tacrolimus exposure in kidney transplanted patients using machine learning
Ability to influence a situation	Mastering and coping in practical health context	Use of phantoms
	Co-creation processes for innovation of assistive technology	Considering elderly people as experts of their own lives
	Developing understandable AI models that can be used in health practice	Interdisciplinary collaboration between medical professionals and AI experts is essential for the successful implementation
	Avoiding misunderstandings	Different terminologies and methodologies used by AI experts and healthcare professionals
	Co-designing new artifacts in health and technology	Construction of low-cost phantoms

Table 1.
Pattern matching analysis of salutogenic concepts in health and technology.

discussing, collaborating, and delivering healthcare services in line with users' needs. Health technology can be seen from interdisciplinary perspectives, like a boundary object [28] where several participants have an interest in a topic from different motivations. Visual technology can be used for common understanding, such as developing understandable AI models that can be used in health practice. This can contribute to co-creation processes for technology innovation. Globalization in health research and education can contribute to a wider perspective [17] for the community to promote collaboration between universities and stakeholders from private and public organizations. Performing in health and technology can be related to interdisciplinary collaboration to improve diagnostics and patient treatment and promote health. Mastering and coping in practical health context can be achieved by learning to use advanced technology and by connecting technologically based health services with people's needs. Finally, experiences can contribute to co-designing new artifacts in health and technology.

4.1 Educational perspectives

The identified collaborative concepts can be related to educational perspectives for group work. In this study, it has relevance to problem-based learning [27], because collaboration with external partners from working life is recommended for higher education innovation systems [17].

In a course that brings together students from diverse backgrounds, it is essential to focus on the most important aspects that foster interdisciplinary understanding and collaboration. To ensure that all students have a good understanding of the core concepts, several aspects can be emphasized.

Common language and interdisciplinary communication are needed. This can develop a shared vocabulary and understanding of key terms and concepts from both the health and technology fields. Encouraging open communication and active listening can facilitate effective interdisciplinary dialog. Relevant applications and case studies can present examples of successful technology in healthcare. Students can discuss the challenges, methodologies, and interdisciplinary collaboration required in these cases, which will help students understand the practical relevance of their learning. Through problem-solving and critical thinking, students can be encouraged to apply their knowledge and skills to solve interdisciplinary problems. This can be done through group projects, case studies, or simulations, where students from diverse backgrounds collaborate and contribute their expertise to address healthcare challenges.

Students should have a good understanding of the most important core concepts and aspects by learning foundational concepts from several fields. Gradually they can build on these foundations with more complex topics, such as applying machine learning algorithms to predict patient outcomes or personalizing treatment plans. Peer learning and collaboration can be strengthened by organizing interdisciplinary group projects that address actual healthcare challenges, such as designing a mobile app for remote patient monitoring or creating a diagnostic tool for early disease detection. Students can be encouraged to share their expertise and learn from each other, fostering a collaborative environment. Providing constructive feedback will help students improve their understanding and address any misconceptions.

By focusing on these important aspects and employing effective pedagogical strategies, educators can create a learning environment that supports interdisciplinary understanding and collaboration, preparing students to contribute meaningfully to the rapidly evolving fields of technology in healthcare.

4.2 A salutogenic perspective in technology and health

A conclusive remark is that the salutogenic perspective applied in this study contributes to a broader and global theoretical framework based on existing literature on salutogenic approaches in public health [5] that can include concepts such as to collaborate with medical equipment, including user journey for designing better health services, and to deliver community health care services in line with users' needs through dialog and reflexivity. Further concepts include co-designing new artifacts in health and technology, stimulating mastering and coping in practical health contexts, and promoting globalization in health research and education.

The study contributes with a case study relevant to higher innovation systems globally [17]. An interdisciplinary understanding of a sense of coherence as described in this study can strengthen the collaboration between professionals and students in health and technology. The results of the current case study show also the potential for replication of the approach in different sites in various countries.

Author details

Arild Berg[1*], Safora Johansen[1], Anne Lund[1], Michael Alexander Riegler[2] and Jorunn Marie Andersen[1]

1 OsloMet – Oslo Metropolitan University, Oslo, Norway

2 OsloMet – Oslo Metropolitan University and SimulaMet, Oslo, Norway

*Address all correspondence to: arild.berg@oslomet.no

References

[1] Greenhalgh T, Jackson C, Shaw S, Janamian T. Achieving research impact through co-creation in community-based health services: Literature review and case study. Milbank Quarterly. 2016;**94**(2):392-429

[2] WHO. Medical devices. 2007. Available from: https://www.who.int/teams/health-product-policy-and-standards/assistive-and-medical-technology/medical-devices

[3] WHO. Assistive technology. 2007 Available from: https://www.who.int/teams/health-product-policy-and-standards/assistive-and-medical-technology/assistive-technology

[4] Hummelvoll JK. In: Dahl TE, editor. Helt - ikke stykkevis og delt: psykiatrisk sykepleie og psykisk helse. 7th ed. Oslo: Gyldendal akademisk; 2012

[5] Lindström B, Eriksson M. Contextualizing salutogenesis and Antonovsky in public health development. Health Promotion International. 2006;**21**(3):238-244

[6] Kuhn TS. The Structure of Scientific Revolutions. 2nd ed. Chicago: University of Chicago Press; 1970

[7] Askheim OP. Samproduksjon som velferdssektorens kinderegg. Tidsskrift for Omsorgsforskning. 2016;**2**(1):24-36

[8] Mohammed Ali A, Hogg P, Johansen S, England A. Construction and validation of a low cost paediatric pelvis phantom. European Journal of Radiology. 2018;**108**:84-91

[9] Nielsen LM, Berg A, Haakonsen P, Lysebo M, Lutnæs E. Education for new practice i – Technology, design and sustainability across professions. Forma. 2020;**13**(6):1-6

[10] European Commission, Directorate-General for Research and Innovation, LAB – FAB – APP – Investing in the European future we want: report of the independent High Level Group on maximising the impact of EU research & innovation programmes. Brussels: Publications Office; 2017

[11] Berg A, Groth C, Medola F, Sellen K. Co-creation of interdisciplinary design educations. In: Proceedings of the DRS LEARN X DESIGN 2021 6th International Conference for Design Education Researchers 24-26 September 2021 Jinan, China Engaging with Challenges in Design Education: Shandong University of Art & Design. Jinan, China: Design Research Society; 2021;**2**;476-478

[12] Antonovsky A. The structure and properties of the sense of coherence scale. Social Science & Medicine. 1993;**36**(6):725-733

[13] Mittelmark MB, Sagy S, Eriksson M, Bauer GF, Pelikan JM, Lindström B, et al. The Handbook of Salutogenesis. Cham (CH): Springer; 2017

[14] Abbott A. The System of Professions: An Essay on the Division of Expert Labor. Chicago: University of Chicago Press; 1988

[15] Vik E. Helseprofesjoners samhandling – en litteraturstudie. Tidsskrift for velferdsforskning. 2018;**21**(2):119-147

[16] Axelsson R, Axelsson SB. Integration and collaboration in public health-a

conceptual framework. The International Journal of Health Planning and Management. 2006;**21**(1):75-88

[17] Cai Y, Ramis Ferrer B, Luis Martinez Lastra J. Building University-Industry Co-Innovation Networks in Transnational Innovation Ecosystems: Towards a Transdisciplinary Approach of Integrating Social Sciences and Artificial Intelligence. In: Sustainability. Basel, Switzerland. 2019;**11**(17):4633

[18] Forsberg E-M, Thorstensen E, Dias Casagrande F, Holthe T, Halvorsrud L, Lund A, et al. Is RRI a new R&I logic? A reflection from an integrated RRI project. Journal of Responsible Technology. 2021;**5**:100007

[19] Yin RK. Case Study Research : Design and Methods. Vol. XIV. Thousand Oaks, Calif: Sage; 2009. p. 219

[20] Maxwell JA. Qualitative Research Design : An Interactive Approach. Thousand Oaks. Vol. XIV. Calif: Sage Publications; 2005. p. 175

[21] Gadamer HG. Truth and Method. London: Sheed and Ward; 1979

[22] Ihde D. Expanding Hermeneutics: Visualism in Science. Evanston, Ill: Northwestern University Press; 1998

[23] Repper J, Breeze J. User and carer involvement in the training and education of health professionals: A review of the literature. International Journal of Nursing Studies. 2007;**44**(3):511-519

[24] Daykin N, Byrne E, Soteriou T, O'Connor S. The impact of art, design and environment in mental healthcare: A systematic review of the literature. Journal of the Royal Society for the Promotion of Health. 2008;**128**(2):85-94

[25] Medola FO, Sandnes FE, Ferrari ALM, Rodrigues ACT. Strategies for Developing Students' Empathy and Awareness for the Needs of People with Disabilities: Contributions to Design Education. Studies in Health Technology and Informatics. 2018;**256**:137-147

[26] Westerveld E. The project excellence model®: Linking success criteria and critical success factors. International Journal of Project Management. 2003;**21**(6):411-418

[27] Scott KS. An integrative framework for problem-based learning and action learning: Promoting evidence-based design and evaluation in leadership development. Human Resource Development Review. 2017;**16**(1):3-34

[28] Star SL, Griesemer JR. Institutional ecology, 'Translations' and boundary objects: Amateurs and professionals in Berkeley's Museum of Vertebrate Zoology, 1907-39. Social Studies of Science. 1989;**19**(3):387-420

[29] Morassaei S, Di Prospero L, Ringdalen E, Olsen SS, Korsell A, Erler D, et al. A survey to explore the psychological impact of the COVID-19 pandemic on radiation therapists in Norway and Canada: A tale of two countries. Journal of Medical Radiation Sciences. 2021;**68**(4):407-417

[30] Hocking C, Whiteford GE. Introduction to Critical Perspectives in Occupational Science. Oxford, UK: Wiley-Blackwell; 2012. pp. 1-7

[31] Holthe T, Halvorsrud L, Lund A. Digital Assistive Technology to Support Everyday Living in Community-Dwelling Older Adults with Mild Cognitive Impairment and Dementia. Clinical Interventions in Aging. 2022;**17**:519-544

[32] Lowes L, Hulatt I. Involving Service Users in Health and Social Care Research. London: Routledge; 2005

[33] Lund A, Holthe T, Halvorsrud L, Karterud D, Johannessen AF, Lovett HM, et al. Involving older adults in technology research and development discussions through dialogue cafés. Research Involvement and Engagement. 2021;7(1):26

[34] Storås AM, Åsberg A, Halvorsen P, Riegler MA, Strümke I. Predicting Tacrolimus Exposure in Kidney Transplanted Patients Using Machine Learning. 2022 IEEE 35th International Symposium on Computer-Based Medical Systems (CBMS). 2022:21-23

[35] World Health O. WHO Laboratory Manual for the Examination and Processing of Human Semen. 5th ed. Geneva: World Health Organization; 2010

[36] Haugen TB, Hicks SA, Witczak O, Andersen JM, Björndahl L, Riegler MA. P–104 assessment of sperm motility according to WHO classification using convolutional neural networks. Human Reproduction. Oxford. 2021;**36**; i183-i184 (Supplement_1)

[37] Risnes M, Mellema M, Pinto-Orellana MA, Sherkat H. Enhancement of collaboration in the early stage of an interdisciplinary engineering and design project: mapping group dynamics. In: Bohemia E, Kovacevic A, Buck L, Brisco R, Evans D, Grierson H, et al., editors. DS 95: Proceedings of the 21st International Conference on Engineering and Product Design Education (E&PDE 2019), University of Strathclyde, Glasgow 12th -13th September 2019. Towards a New Innovation Landscape. 21: The Design Society; 2019. p. 6.

[38] Risnes M, Korostynska O, Mirtaheri P, Berg A. The role of human experience when making sense of brain monitoring: An interdisciplinary case study to assess wearable, non-invasive, brain-monitoring devices for rehabilitation. Journal of Responsible Innovation. 2023;**10**:1-20

Chapter 6

Evolving Role of Social Media in Health Promotion

Rajshri Roy and Jessica Malloy

Abstract

Social media has become integral to our daily lives and has transformed how people communicate and share information. It has also emerged as a powerful tool in health promotion and health policy. Social media can be used to raise awareness about health issues and promote healthy behaviours. Health organisations and advocates can use social media to share educational content, infographics and videos to promote health awareness. Social media can be used to motivate and support behaviour change. Health organisations and advocates can use social media to provide real-time support and encouragement, share success stories and offer tips and advice. Social media can also help policymakers engage with communities and stakeholders. Social media can build trust and strengthen relationships by sharing information, asking for feedback, and responding to comments and concerns. By analysing social media conversations, health organisations and policymakers can better understand public opinion and use that information to inform policy decisions. Social media can also be a powerful platform for advocacy and activism to raise awareness about health-related issues, organise events and campaigns, and mobilise support for policy change.

Keywords: social media, health promotion, health education, health policy, social media communication, health information

1. Introduction

Social media platforms have become an integral part of our daily lives [1]. From Facebook to Instagram, Twitter to TikTok, we use social media to connect with family and friends, stay up-to-date with news and current events, and share our experiences and opinions. Social media has also become a powerful tool for health promotion. By leveraging the vast reach and influence of social media, healthcare professionals can engage with patients and the general public, disseminate health information, and promote healthy behaviours [2].

Social media plays a critical role in health promotion and health policy by raising awareness, facilitating behaviour change, engaging communities, gathering data and promoting advocacy and activism [3]. Social media has become an increasingly important tool for health promotion and policy changes by providing new opportunities for reaching and engaging with diverse audiences [4]. In recent years, social media has emerged as a powerful tool for communication and information-sharing. With the proliferation of social media platforms, individuals and organisations have an unprecedented ability to connect and share health-related messages with large audiences [5]. As a result, social media has become an increasingly important component of health promotion efforts [6].

The evolving role of social media in health promotion is the focus of this book chapter. We will examine the ways in which social media has been used to promote health and prevent disease, as well as its potential benefits and limitations. We will explore the different types of health-related content that are shared on social media, including health information, health behaviours, and social support. Additionally, we will discuss the challenges and ethical considerations associated with using social media for health promotion, including issues of privacy, accuracy, and accessibility.

2. Health promotion and disease prevention

Social media provides an accessible and convenient platform for sharing health information with large audiences. Health organisations and professionals use social media to disseminate information on a wide range of topics, including disease prevention, healthy lifestyles, and treatments [7–9]. Health promotion has come a long way since the days of print brochures and public service announcements. Ruppel and Rains discuss the opportunities and challenges of health communication in the age of social media [10]. The authors argue that social media offers new and innovative ways for healthcare professionals to engage with audiences through visually appealing content such as videos, infographics, and other multimedia. With the advent of social media, health promotion has become more interactive, engaging, and accessible. Social media platforms offer a range of tools and features that enable healthcare professionals to connect with patients and the general public in new and innovative ways. A literature review by Coughlin and colleagues explores the use of smartphone applications for promoting healthy diet and nutrition [11]. The authors discuss the use of social media platforms such as Instagram and Pinterest to share visually appealing content related to healthy eating, such as recipes and food photos. For example, social media platforms allow healthcare professionals to create and share videos, infographics, and other visually appealing content that can help educate and engage audiences. Maher and colleagues discuss the potential of social media and mobile applications for health promotion and disease prevention [12]. The authors argue that social media platforms offer a range of tools and features that enable healthcare professionals to create and share visually appealing content, such as videos and infographics, that can help educate and engage audiences.

2.1 Influencer marketing

Influencer marketing can be a powerful tool for health organisations, advocates, and policymakers in health promotion and policy changes. Health organisations, advocates and policymakers can collaborate with influencers in their respective fields to spread important health messages and promote healthy behaviours [13]. Influencers can share evidence-based information and use their platforms to amplify health promotion campaigns [4]. They can engage with health influencers in policy discussions to gather insights and opinions from their perspectives. This can help to inform policy decisions and create more effective health interventions. Insights from influencer marketing campaigns can be used to inform policy changes. Chu et al. discuss the potential of social media influencers for health promotion, including their role in policy discussions [14]. The authors argue that influencers can provide valuable insights and opinions from their perspectives that can inform policy decisions and create more effective health interventions.

For example, policymakers can analyse the data from social media campaigns to identify trends in health behaviours and preferences, which can then inform policy decisions [15]. They can partner with influencers to advocate for policy changes that promote public health. Influencers can use their platforms to raise awareness about important health issues and mobilise to support policy changes. Influencer marketing can target specific populations at higher risk for certain health conditions or who may be harder to reach through traditional health communication channels. Mantzarlis discusses the potential of influencer marketing campaigns to impact public health, including their role in advocating for policy changes that promote public health [16].

By partnering with influencers with large followings within these populations, they can reach a wider audience and promote healthy behaviours [17, 18]. Taylor et al. reviewed the literature on influencer marketing and discussed its potential for promoting healthy behaviours and driving policy changes [19]. The authors argue that influencer marketing can be a valuable tool for targeting specific populations at higher risk for certain health conditions or who may be harder to reach through traditional health communication channels. Overall, influencer marketing can be a valuable tool for health organisations and policymakers to promote healthy behaviours and drive policy changes. By leveraging the reach and influence of influencers, they can reach a wider audience and have a greater impact on public health.

2.2 User-generated content

User-generated content (UGC) refers to any content that is created and shared by users of online platforms, such as social media [20]. Health organisations, advocates, and policymakers can use UGC to support their health promotion and policy change efforts in several ways. UGC can be used to amplify health messages by sharing user-generated posts that align with a particular health promotion campaign or policy initiative [21]. By sharing UGC, health promoters can demonstrate that their messages resonate with real people and help raise engagement and reach. UGC can be used to engage with communities by inviting users to share their experiences and opinions about health-related topics. This can help to build trust and create ownership in health promotion efforts and policy changes [22].

By involving users in the creative process, health organisations, advocacy, and policymakers can ensure that their campaigns resonate with the intended audience and increase the likelihood of success. UGC can also be used to collect data on health behaviours and attitudes. By analysing user-generated content, health organisations and policymakers can gain insights into the needs and preferences of different populations and use this information to inform policy decisions and health promotion efforts [23]. A study by Abroms et al. analysed popular smartphone apps for smoking cessation and found that those that incorporated user-generated content were more likely to be effective in helping users quit smoking [24]. Litchman et al. described a user-centred design process for developing a mobile health website for diabetes prevention and management [25]. The authors argue that involving users in the design process can help ensure that the website is usable and appealing to the intended audience. Additionally, by tracking user-generated content related to health behaviours and policies, health organisations and policymakers can identify areas where compliance may be low and target interventions to improve adherence [5]. UGC can be valuable for health organisations and policymakers in health promotion and policy change efforts. By leveraging the creativity and insights of users, they can increase engagement, build trust, and create more effective health interventions [26].

2.3 Social media monitoring

Social media can be used to collect data on health behaviours, attitudes, and perceptions [27, 28]. This can help researchers and health organisations better understand the needs and preferences of different populations and design more effective interventions [5]. Social media monitoring can benefit health organisations, advocates, and policymakers in health promotion and policy changes. Social media monitoring can be used to identify emerging health trends and concerns among different populations.

By analysing social media conversations related to health, organisations and policymakers can identify areas of concern and respond with appropriate health interventions [29–31]. It can be used to monitor public sentiment related to health issues and policy changes [32]. This can help organisations and policymakers gauge public support for different policy initiatives and adjust their strategies accordingly. Social media conversations related to health issues and policy changes can be monitored, and organisations and policymakers can engage with stakeholders, answer questions, and address concerns in real time [33].

The effectiveness of health promotion campaigns can be evaluated using social media monitoring. Public health organisations and policymakers can identify what works and what does not by analysing social media engagement and sentiment related to specific campaigns and adjusting their strategies accordingly. Social media conversations about health behaviours and policies can identify areas where compliance may be low and target interventions to improve adherence [34]. Social media monitoring can be a powerful tool for health organisations, advocates, and policymakers in health promotion and policy changes. By leveraging the real-time insights social media monitoring provides, they can identify emerging health trends, engage with stakeholders, and evaluate the effectiveness of health promotion campaigns and policy changes.

2.4 Online health communities

Social media platforms can facilitate the formation of communities centred around health issues. These communities can provide social support, encouragement, and a sense of belonging to people with similar health concerns [35–38].

Online health communities can benefit health organisations, advocates, and policymakers in health promotion and policy changes, as they can support health education efforts by providing a platform for health organisations, advocates and policymakers to share evidence-based information about health and wellness [3]. Members of the community can also share their own experiences and knowledge to promote health literacy [39, 40]. Engaging with community members openly and transparently can build relationships and create a sense of shared ownership in health promotion efforts and policy changes.

Public health organisations and policymakers can use these communities to gather insights into the needs and preferences of different populations and use this information to inform policy decisions and health promotion efforts [5]. Online health communities can be used to support advocacy efforts by providing a platform

DOI: http://dx.doi.org/10.5772/intechopen.111967

for community members to share their stories and advocate for policy changes that promote public health. These communities can be used to engage with advocates and identify areas where policy changes may be needed. Furthermore, by connecting individuals with others who have similar experiences, health organisations, and policymakers can help to improve mental and emotional health outcomes and promote positive health behaviours.

3. Different types of health-related content

Social media has become a powerful tool for sharing health-related information and engaging in health behaviours. Health-related content on social media can be broadly categorised into three main types: health information, health behaviours, and social support.

Health information refers to any content related to health or healthcare. This can include information about medical conditions, treatments, medications, and preventative health measures. Social media platforms like Twitter and Facebook are often used to share health information, and many health organisations have established a social media presence to disseminate accurate and up-to-date health information to their followers [41–43]. Individuals may also share health information on their personal social media accounts, either to raise awareness about a particular health issue or to seek advice from their social networks.

Health behaviours refer to the actions individuals take to maintain or improve their health [44]. Examples of health behaviours include exercise, healthy eating, and getting enough sleep. Social media can be used to promote and encourage healthy behaviours, either through direct messaging or through the sharing of motivational content [45]. Many fitness influencers have built a following on social media platforms like Instagram by sharing their own healthy lifestyle habits and encouraging their followers to adopt similar habits.

Social support refers to the emotional and practical support individuals receive from their social networks [46]. Social media can be a powerful tool for providing social support, particularly for individuals with chronic health conditions [47–49]. Online support groups and forums allow individuals to connect with others who are going through similar experiences, providing a sense of community and shared understanding. Social media can also be used to connect individuals with health professionals or other resources that can provide additional support.

In summary, social media plays a significant role in the sharing of health-related content. Health information, health behaviours, and social support are three main types of content that are commonly shared on social media platforms. By providing access to accurate and up-to-date health information, promoting healthy behaviours, and facilitating social support, social media has the potential to positively impact individuals' health and well-being. However, it is important to recognise the limitations and potential risks of social media use, including the spread of misinformation and the potential for social media to exacerbate existing health disparities.

4. Key benefits and challenges of social media in health promotion

See **Table 1**.

Benefits	Challenges
Increased reach: Social media has a vast user base, which provides an opportunity to reach a large and diverse audience with health messages.	**Lack of regulation:** Social media is largely unregulated, which can lead to the spread of inaccurate or misleading health information.
Cost-effective: Social media is a relatively low-cost way to disseminate health information and promote behaviour change.	**Privacy concerns:** Social media platforms collect a vast amount of user data, raising concerns about privacy and the potential misuse of personal information.
Accessible: Social media is easily accessible to most people with an internet connection, making it an effective way to reach underserved populations.	**Limited engagement:** While social media can be an effective way to reach a large audience, engagement and behaviour change are not guaranteed.
Interactive: Social media allows for two-way communication and interaction between health organisations and their audiences, which can improve engagement and promote behaviour change.	**Digital divide:** Not everyone has access to social media or the digital literacy skills required to use it effectively, which can limit the reach of health promotion efforts.
Analytics: By tracking social media metrics, health advocates can get a much clearer sense of how their health promotion campaign is performing on social media. This can help make informed decisions about where to focus efforts and how to optimise messaging to achieve your desired outcomes.	**Algorithms:** Social media platforms regularly update their algorithms in order to improve user experience and keep up with changing trends. Ever-changing social media algorithms can be a challenge for organisations that are trying to measure the success of their health promotion campaigns or increase the reach of their content.

Table 1.
Potential benefits and challenges associated with using social media for health promotion.

5. Social media's impact on health education and literacy

While social media has many benefits when it comes to health promotion, there are also several challenges and limitations. Notably, social media can be a source of misinformation, as anyone can share information on social media, regardless of its accuracy. This can lead to confusion and mistrust among patients and those seeking health advice online [50, 51].

Through the seeking and sharing of information, social media can have a significant impact on health education and literacy [52]. Social media has resulted in greater access to health information, allowing individuals to educate themselves on health topics, as well as greater engagement in health education [5]. As individuals participate in online discussions and connect with others who are interested in similar health topics, the quality of information shared can greatly influence health knowledge.

Using social media as a tool for health promotion acts to improve the quality of health information online, as well as the likelihood of encountering evidence-based guidance and advice. The voices of health professionals and the presence of healthcare organisations on social media are required to dilute misinformation in the digital health space, where evidence-based information can be difficult to source [53].

Healthcare organisations should take advantage of the greater transparency that social media allows in health education, whereby the sharing of information about their services and outcomes allows patients to make informed decisions about their healthcare [7]. This plays an important role in autonomy and trust in healthcare services and providers.

As well as transparency, social media has also allowed for greater accountability in health education. Individuals can hold healthcare providers and organisations accountable for the accuracy and quality of their health information. Similarly, organisations can bring awareness to misinformation and offer guidance to individuals as to how it can be identified and avoided.

6. Effective strategies for using social media platforms in health promotion

See **Table 2**.

Social media platform	Strategy
Facebook	Post updates, articles, infographics, and videos related to health promotion campaigns or initiatives. Engage with the audience by responding to comments and messages. Use Facebook ads to target the desired audience.
Twitter	Use hashtags relevant to health promotion campaigns or initiatives in the tweets. Tweet links to articles, infographics, and videos related to campaign or initiative. Engage with the audience by responding to tweets and direct messages.
Instagram	Post images and videos related to campaigns or initiatives. Use hashtags relevant to campaign or initiative in posts. Use Instagram Stories and Live to provide updates and engage with the audience. Collaborate with influencers to reach a wider audience. Encourage positive dialogue in comment sections. Create a sense of community.
YouTube	Post videos related to health promotion campaigns or initiatives. Use keywords in video titles and descriptions to improve visibility. Collaborate with other YouTubers and organisations to reach a wider audience. Utilise YouTube Shorts for brevity and engagement.
LinkedIn	Post articles and updates related to the health promotion campaign or initiative. Engage with the audience by responding to comments and messages. Use LinkedIn ads to target the desired audience.
TikTok	Create short videos that are informative and engaging. Use hashtags relevant to the health campaign or initiative in the videos. Collaborate with other TikTokers and organisations to reach a wider audience. Use humour and trending songs or audio to boost content and relate to audiences.

Table 2.
Social media strategies for health promotion.

7. Success stories and key lessons: harnessing the power of social media for health promotion

There have been several notable success stories and lessons learned from health promotion initiatives that have effectively utilised social media. Some key examples include:

1. **#ThisGirlCan Campaign:** The #ThisGirlCan campaign launched by Sport England [54] and also implemented in Australia [55] is a prime example of a successful health promotion campaign on social media. It aimed to encourage women of all shapes, sizes, and abilities to participate in physical activities. The campaign used authentic and empowering images and videos of real women, which

resonated with the target audience and resulted in widespread engagement and positive behavioural change.

2. **Smoking Cessation Campaigns:** Social media has proven to be an effective platform for promoting smoking cessation. Campaigns like the National Health Service's "Stoptober" [56] and the American Cancer Society's "Great American Smokeout" [57] have utilised social media to provide support, resources, and encouragement to individuals trying to quit smoking. These campaigns have successfully reached large audiences, provided relevant information, and facilitated peer support, leading to increased quitting attempts and successful smoking cessation outcomes.

3. **Mental health awareness:** Social media has played a significant role in raising awareness and reducing the stigma surrounding mental health. Initiatives like the "Bell Let's Talk" campaign in Canada [58] and the "It's Okay to Not Be Okay" campaign by mental health organisations [59] have utilised social media platforms to encourage open conversations about mental health, share personal stories, provide mental health resources, and connect individuals with support services. These campaigns have been instrumental in increasing awareness, reducing stigma, and promoting mental health support-seeking behaviours.

4. **Disease awareness and fundraising:** Social media has been instrumental in raising awareness and funds for various health conditions. Movements like the ALS Ice Bucket Challenge [60] and the Breast Cancer Awareness Month campaigns [61] have gained significant traction on social media, reaching millions of people and raising substantial funds for research and support services.

8. Conclusions

Overall, this chapter provides a comprehensive overview of the evolving role of social media in health promotion. By understanding the potential benefits and limitations of social media in this context, we can develop effective strategies for using these platforms to promote health and prevent disease. Lessons learned from success stories of health promotion using social media include the importance of authentic and relatable content, utilising engaging visuals, leveraging user-generated content, fostering community and peer support, and utilising influencers or advocates to amplify the message. It is crucial to understand the target audience, tailor the content to the platform and user behaviour, and actively monitor and respond to user engagement to ensure the success of health promotion initiatives on social media.

Conflict of interest

The authors declare no conflict of interest.

Author details

Rajshri Roy* and Jessica Malloy
Department of Nutrition and Dietetics, University of Auckland, Auckland, New Zealand

*Address all correspondence to: r.roy@auckland.ac.nz

References

[1] Statista. Number of Social Media Users Worldwide from 2010 to 2026. 2021. Available from: https://www.statista.com/statistics/278414/number-of-worldwide-social-network-users/

[2] Lee J, Sun C, Lee JK, Jiang S. The impact of social media on healthcare professionals and patients: A scoping review. Journal of Medical Internet Research. 2017;**19**(8):e282. DOI: 10.2196/jmir.7627

[3] Stellefson M, Paige SR, Chaney BH, Chaney JD. Evolving role of social media in health promotion: Updated responsibilities for health education specialists. International Journal of Environmental Research and Public Health. 2020;**17**(4):1153. DOI: 10.3390/ijerph17041153

[4] Klassen KM, Borleis ES, Brennan L, Reid M, TA MC, Lim MS. What people "like": Analysis of social media strategies used by food industry brands, lifestyle brands, and health promotion organizations on Facebook and Instagram. Journal of Medical Internet Research. 2018;**20**(6):e10227. DOI: 10.2196/10227

[5] Chen J, Wang Y. Social media use for health purposes: Systematic review. Journal of Medical Internet Research. 2021;**23**(5):e17917. DOI: 10.2196/17917

[6] De Leo G, Brivio E, Corno G, Giorgi I. Social media and healthcare: An overview. Journal of Public Health Research. 2019;**8**(2):1548. DOI: 10.4081/jphr.2019.1548

[7] Smailhodzic E, Hooijsma W, Boonstra A, et al. Social media use in healthcare: A systematic review of effects on patients and on their relationship with healthcare professionals. BMC Health Services Research. 2016;**16**:442. DOI: 10.1186/s12913-016-1691-0

[8] Pachankis JE, Lelutiu-Weinberger C, Golub SA, Parsons JT. Developing an online health intervention for young gay and bisexual men. AIDS and Behavior. 2013;**17**(9):2986-2998. DOI: 10.1007/s10461-013-0499-8

[9] Moorhead S, Hazlett D, Harrison L, Carroll J, Irwin A, Hoving C. A new dimension of health care: Systematic review of the uses, benefits, and limitations of social media for health communication. Journal of Medical Internet Research. 2013;**15**(4):e85. DOI: 10.2196/jmir.1933

[10] Ruppel EK, Rains SA. Health communication in the age of social media: Opportunities and challenges for public health. Journal of Public Health Management & Practice. 2018;**24**(6):510-516. DOI: 10.1097/PHH.0000000000000807

[11] Coughlin SS, Whitehead M, Sheats JQ, Mastromonico J, Hardy D, Smith SA. Smartphone applications for promoting healthy diet and nutrition: A literature review. Jacobs Journal of Food and Nutrition. 2015;**2**(3):021

[12] Maher C, Ryan J, Kernot J, Podsiadly J, Keenihan S. Social media and applications to health promotion and disease prevention. Digit Health. 2016;**9**:50-55. DOI: 10.1016/j.copsyc.2015.10.021

[13] Kostygina G, Tran H, Binns S, Szczypka G, Emery S, Vallone D, et al. Boosting health campaign reach and engagement through use of social media influencers and memes. Social

Media + Society. 2020;**6**(2):1-12. DOI: 10.1177/2056305120912475

[14] Zou W, Zhang WJ, Tang L. What do social media influencers say about health? A theory-driven content analysis of top ten health influencers' posts on Sina Weibo. Journal of Health Communication. 2 Jan 2021;**26**(1):1-1

[15] Simonofski A, Fink J, Burnay C. Supporting policy-making with social media and e-participation platforms data: A policy analytics framework. Government Information Quarterly. 2021;**38**(3):101590. DOI: 10.1016/j.giq.2021.101590

[16] Mantzarlis A. PLOS Blogs. Can Influencer Marketing Campaigns Impact Public Health? [Internet]. 2018. Available from: https://blogs.plos.org/publichealth/2018/04/16/can-influencer-marketing-campaigns-impact-public-health/

[17] Bonnevie E, Smith SM, Kummeth C, Goldbarg J, Smyser J. Social media influencers can be used to deliver positive information about the flu vaccine: Findings from a multi-year study. Health Education Research. 2021;**36**(3):286-294. DOI: 10.1093/her/cyab018

[18] Schillinger D, Chittamuru D, Ramírez S. From "infodemics" to health promotion: A novel framework for the role of social media in public health. American Journal of Public Health. 2020;**110**(9):1393-1396. DOI: 10.2105/AJPH.2020.305746

[19] Taylor K, Silver L, Huang M. Influencer marketing: A review and research agenda. Journal of Advertising. 2020;**49**(1):34-49. DOI: 10.1080/00913367.2019.1684559

[20] Wyrwoll C. User-generated content. In: Social Media. Wiesbaden: Springer Vieweg; 2014. DOI: 10.1007/978-3-658-06984-1_2

[21] Hether J, Calabrese CJ. Beyond #liking: Inspiring user-generated content for health promotion. In: Kim J, Song H, editors. Technology and Health: Promoting Attitude and Behavior Change. Elsevier; 2020. p. 291-312. DOI: 10.1016/B978-0-12-816958-2.00013-7

[22] Cuomo MT, Tortora D, Giordano A, Festa G, Metallo G, Martinelli E. User-generated content in the era of digital well-being: A netnographic analysis in a healthcare marketing context. Psychology and Marketing. 2020;**37**(4):578-587. DOI: 10.1002/mar.21327

[23] Ruppel EK, Rains SA. User-generated content as health communication: A theoretical and empirical overview. Health Communication. 2018;**33**(9):1135-1144. DOI: 10.1080/10410236.2017.1350400

[24] Abroms LC, Lee Westmaas J, Bontemps-Jones J, Ramani R, Mellerson J. A content analysis of popular smartphone apps for smoking cessation. American Journal of Preventive Medicine. 2013;**45**(6):732-736. DOI: 10.1016/j.amepre.2013.07.008

[25] Litchman ML, Rothwell E, Edelman LS, Theeke LA. User-centered design of a mobile health website for the prevention and management of diabetes. Journal of Medical Internet Research. 2015;**17**(9):e207. DOI: 10.2196/jmir.4822

[26] Zhou J, Wan X. How to build network effects on online platforms for mental health. California Management Review. 2022;**64**(4):20-46. DOI: 10.1177/00081256221107421

[27] Lin L, Sidhu TS, Farley S. Using social media for actionable disease surveillance and outbreak management:

A systematic literature review. PLoS One. 2018;**13**(12):e0208401. DOI: 10.1371/journal.pone.020840

[28] Ahmed W, Bath PA, Demartini G. Using social media for health research: Methodological and ethical considerations for recruitment and intervention delivery. Digit Health. 2019;**5**:2055207619867226. DOI: 10.1177/2055207619867226

[29] Bello-Orgaz G, Hernandez-Castro J, Camacho D. A survey of social web mining applications for disease outbreak detection. In: Camacho D, Braubach L, Venticinque S, Badica C, editors. Intelligent Distributed Computing VIII. Studies in Computational Intelligence. 570. Berlin: Springer-Verlag; 2015. pp. 345-356. DOI: 10.1007/978-3-319-10422-5_36

[30] Allen C, Tsou M-H, Aslam A, Nagel A, Gawron J-M. Applying GIS and machine learning methods to twitter data for multiscale surveillance of influenza. PLoS One. 2016;**11**(7):e0157734. DOI: 10.1371/journal.pone.0157734

[31] Pilipiec P, Samsten I, Bota A. Surveillance of communicable diseases using social media: A systematic review. PLoS One. 2023;**18**(2):e0282101. DOI: 10.1371/journal.pone.0282101

[32] Stieglitz S, Dang-Xuan L. Emotions and information diffusion in social media - Sentiment of microblogs and sharing behavior. Journal of Management Information Systems. 2013;**29**:217-248. DOI: 10.2753/MIS0742-1222290408

[33] Lin Y, Huang SL, Sun Y. Applying social media analytics to investigate the effectiveness of smoking cessation campaigns. Health Informatics Journal. 2019;**25**(4):1495-1506. DOI: 10.1177/1460458218769065

[34] Bennett GG, Glasgow RE. The delivery of public health interventions via the internet: Actualizing their potential. Annual Review of Public Health. 2009;**30**(1):273-292. DOI: 10.1146/annurev.publhealth.031308.100235

[35] Hwang KO, Ottenbacher AJ, Green AP, Cannon-Diehl MR, Richardson O, Bernstam EV, et al. Social support in an internet weight loss community. International Journal of Medical Informatics. 2010;**79**(1):5-13. DOI: 10.1016/j.ijmedinf.2009.10.003

[36] White M, Dorman SM. Receiving social support online: Implications for health education. Health Education Research. 2001;**16**(6):693-707. DOI: 10.1093/her/16.6.693

[37] Wright KB, Bell SB, Wright KB, Bell SB. Health-related support groups on the internet: Linking empirical findings to social support and computer-mediated communication theory. Journal of Health Psychology. 2003;**8**(1):39-54. DOI: 10.1177/1359105303008001429

[38] Pfeil U, Zaphiris P, Wilson S. Online support communities for older people: Network patterns and characteristics of computer-mediated communication. In: Proceedings of Workshop Enhancing Interaction Spaces by Social Media for the Elderly. Vienna, Austria: European Conference on Computer-Supported Cooperative Work (ECSCW); Sep 2009:7-11

[39] Lu X, Zhang R. Association between eHealth literacy in online health communities and patient adherence: Cross-sectional questionnaire study. Journal of Management Information Research. 2021;**23**(9):e14908. DOI: 10.2196/14908

[40] Coulson NS, Buchanan H, Aubeeluck A. Social support in

cyberspace: A content analysis of communication within a Huntington's disease online support group. Patient Education and Counseling. 2007;**68**(2):173-178. DOI: 10.1016/j.pec.2007.05.016

[41] Shan LC, Panagiotopoulos P, Regan Á, De Brún A, Barnett J, Wall P, et al. Interactive communication with the public: Qualitative exploration of the use of social media by food and health organizations. Journal of Nutrition Education and Behavior. 2015;**47**(1):104-108. DOI: 10.1016/j.jneb.2014.09.004

[42] Ramanadhan S, Mendez SR, Rao M, et al. Social media use by community-based organizations conducting health promotion: A content analysis. BMC Public Health. 2013;**13**:1129. DOI: 10.1186/1471-2458-13-1129

[43] Park H, Rodgers S, Stemmle J. Health organizations' use of facebook for health advertising and promotion. Juvenile Idiopathic Arthritis. 2011;**12**(1):62-77. DOI: 10.1080/15252019.2011.10722191

[44] Short SE, Mollborn S. Social determinants and health behaviors: Conceptual frames and empirical advances. Current Opinion in Psychology. 2015;**5**:78-84. DOI: 10.1016/j.copsyc.2015.05.002

[45] Seiler J, Libby TE, Jackson E, Lingappa JR, Evans WD. Social media-based interventions for health behavior change in low- and middle-income countries: Systematic review. Journal of Medical Internet Research. 2022;**24**(4):e31889. DOI: 10.2196/31889

[46] Zhou ES. Social support. In: Michalos AC, editor. Encyclopedia of Quality of Life and Well-Being Research. Dordrecht: Springer; 2014. DOI: 10.1007/978-94-007-0753-5_2789

[47] Vaingankar JA, van Dam RM, Samari E, Chang S, Seow E, Chua YC, et al. Social media-driven routes to positive mental health among youth: Qualitative enquiry and concept mapping study. JPP. 2022;**5**(1):e32758. DOI: 10.2196/32758

[48] Zhang S, O'Carroll Bantum E, Owen J, Bakken S, Elhadad N. Online cancer communities as informatics intervention for social support: Conceptualization, characterization, and impact. Journal of the American Medical Informatics Association. 2017;**24**(2):451-459. DOI: 10.1093/jamia/ocw093

[49] Coulson NS, Greenwood N. Families affected by childhood cancer: An analysis of the provision of social support within online support groups. Child: Care, Health and Development. 2012;**38**:870-877. DOI: 10.1111/j.1365-2214.2011.01316.x

[50] Krishna A, Thompson TL. Misinformation about health: A review of health communication and misinformation scholarship. The American Behavioral Scientist. 2021;**65**(2):316-332. DOI: 10.1177/0002764219878223

[51] Swire-Thompson B, Lazer D. Public health and online misinformation: Challenges and recommendations. Annual Review of Public Health. 2020;**41**(1):433-451. DOI: 10.1146/annurev-publhealth-040119-094127

[52] Lowry M, Trivedi N, Boyd P, et al. Making decisions about health information on social media: A mouse-tracking study. Cognitive Research. 2022;7:68. DOI: 10.1186/s41235-022-00414-5

[53] Wang Y, McKee M, Torbica A, Stuckler D. Systematic literature review on the spread of health-related misinformation on social media. Social Science & Medicine. 2019;**240**:112552. DOI: 10.1016/j.socscimed.2019.112552

[54] England S. This Girl Can: Campaign Summary. Loughborough, UK: Sport England

[55] Bauman A, McNeil N, Nicholson M, O'Halloran P, Seal E, Randle E, et al. Impact of the first year of the "this girl can" physical activity and sport mass media campaign in Australia. BMC Public Health. 2023;**23**(1):1-9

[56] Brown J, Kotz D, Michie S, Stapleton J, Walmsley M, West R. How effective and cost-effective was the national mass media smoking cessation campaign 'Stoptober'? Drug and Alcohol Dependence. 2014;**135**:52-58

[57] Ayers JW, Westmaas JL, Leas EC, Benton A, Chen Y, Dredze M, et al. Leveraging big data to improve health awareness campaigns: A novel evaluation of the great American smokeout. JMIR Public Health and Surveillance. 2016;**2**(1):e5304

[58] Vido J. A Critical Investigation of Bell Let's Talk

[59] iokn2bok. Mental Health. Available from: https://iokn2bok.org/ [Accessed: May 19, 2023]

[60] Pressgrove G, McKeever BW, Jang SM. What is contagious? Exploring why content goes viral on twitter: A case study of the ALS ice bucket challenge. International Journal of Nonprofit and Voluntary Sector Marketing. 2018;**23**(1):e1586

[61] Jacobsen GD, Jacobsen KH. Health awareness campaigns and diagnosis rates: Evidence from National Breast Cancer Awareness Month. Journal of Health Economics. 2011;**30**(1):55-61

Chapter 7

Health Promotion and Disease Prevention in Botswana

Esther Salang Seloilwe, Kebope Mongie Kealeboga, Joyce V. Khutjwe, Lesedi Mosebetsi and Tebogo T. Mamalelala

Abstract

This chapter discusses health promotion and its usefulness in preventing diseases in Botswana. Document analysis, published and non-published, was conducted to illustrate how health promotion is implemented in Botswana. First, the contextual definition and meaning of health promotion is given, emphasising the cultivation of positive health behaviours in individuals, communities and the nation to prevent numerous health problems and diseases that Botswana faces. Next, health promotion models, programs, strategies and interventions applicable to the Botswana situation and the achievements made were examined. Finally, the chapter concludes by assessing health promotion processes and measures that have enabled people to increase control in improving their health and cultivating a positive health concept through participation and involvement are examined.

Keywords: health promotion, health promotion strategies, disease prevention, Botswana, healthcare

1. Introduction

The Botswana health care system has made significant strides in providing health care services since independence in 1966. The impetus to this realisation was partly due to the health status of the people and the context under which health care delivery was premised. From the onset, Botswana needed to position itself better to offer promotive, preventive and curative care services since most people needed access. Thus, preventive and health-promotive services were imperative. Health promotion and preventive services were also conceptualised before the Alma Ata Declaration on Health for All by 2000 and beyond.

Although a universal concept, health promotion is shaped and influenced by its operative context. Its central tenets focus on individuals' development to take responsibility for their health. From the Botswana perspective, health is a primary responsibility of every individual and the health care provider is responsible for empowering each person to embrace this responsibility.

Many define health promotion differently, but its essence cuts across many healthcare systems. Health promotion is defined as enabling people to increase control over and improve their health [1]. This definition was crystallised at the first International

Conference on Health Promotion in Ottawa in 1986 and became known as the Ottawa Charter. The basic strategies for health promotion identified in the Ottawa Charter are advocacy to boost the factors which encourage health, allowing all people to achieve health equity and mediation through collaboration across all sectors [1]. Since then, the WHO Global Health Promotion Conferences have established and developed the global principles and action areas for health promotion.

According to WHO, the concept of health is particular because it covers the extent to which a group or individuals can fulfil their aspirations and needs on the other hand and evolves with or adapts to the environment on the other [1]. Further, health is seen as a resource for everyday life and not just a life goal. It is a positive concept emphasising social and individual resources and physical capabilities [1]. Thus, health promotion is not just a health issue but goes beyond healthy lifestyles to well-being.

The Ottawa Charter identifies the prerequisites of health promotion as peace, shelter, education, food, income, a stable ecosystem, sustainable resources, social justice and equity. It further pinpoints the action areas as building public health policy, creating a supportive environment, strengthening the country's action, developing personal skills and re-orientating health care delivery services towards prevention of illness and promotion of health, bearing in mind the prevailing contextual conditions [1].

2. Methodology

This chapter analysed and examined the concept of health promotion in Botswana and utilised document review to explore health promotion and disease prevention in Botswana. According to Centres for Disease and Prevention [2], document review "is a way of collecting data by reviewing existing documents". This entailed the review of available Botswana health policies and the different health programs implemented, the Ottawa Charter, and other unpublished documents to gain a contextual understanding of how Botswana promotes health and prevents diseases.

2.1 Analysis, conclusions and interpretations

The following discussion outlines the analysis results, conclusions and inferences on how health promotion and disease prevention are implemented in Botswana. The discussion also examined the fundamental conditions required for health promotion to be implemented successfully. These include but are not limited to how the health care system is organised and the resources, processes, programmes and interventions implemented.

3. Botswana health care system

Two healthcare systems run concurrently in Botswana: Western and traditional healthcare. Every Motswana (a person living in Botswana) has access to traditional health, and only some have access to Western health care. People's beliefs, customs and values influence the selection of which healthcare system to access. The common practice is that people exhaust the traditional healthcare services before consulting Western healthcare, especially if one suffers from an illness that needs to be clearly understood. Therefore, healthcare providers must take into cognisance the operations of these systems and fully comprehend the belief system of the people they serve to strike a balance between the two health systems.

3.1 Western health care

At independence in 1966, Botswana inherited a largely curative, hospital-based health care delivery system from the British, with most of the population without access to services [3]. Therefore, hospital-based health care challenged the government to provide health care for most people, thus necessitating the building of basic health facilities throughout the country. The main objectives were to strengthen the primary health care services, equitably distribute them to all people with more emphasis in the rural areas and improve hospitals to ensure adequate referral services [3]. The emphasis of the health policy N0.1 of 1970 was directed towards preventing more life-threatening health problems such as maternal and child health and combating communicable diseases such as childhood conditions, tuberculosis, and malaria. The policy trend has not changed significantly since its inception, but it has also infused the prevention of non-communicable diseases [4].

The health delivery philosophy in Botswana is to provide quality and affordable health services to Batswana. It is based on a decentralised model, with primary health care being the cornerstone in delivering health services. This system comprises a network of health facilities organised at different levels of sophistication and coverage [1]. Initially, the population and distance guided the infrastructure development [3]. Therefore, a 15-kilometre radius and a population of 500 people were prerequisite criteria [5]. Currently, the population of Botswana is about 2.346,179 million [5]. Health facilities are distributed according to the population and catchment areas they are to serve. It is currently estimated that most of the population lives within 5 km of a health facility [6].

Botswana has 27 health districts comprising the lowest and the highest referral services [7]. The mobile stops or outreach (921) are at the lowest level, where services are generally provided under a tree or at a school. Then follows health posts (351), clinics without beds (206), Clinics with beds (101), 17 primary health hospitals, 15 districts and three referral hospitals at the top [8, 9]. Finally, a teaching hospital at the University of Botswana, a quaternary public health facility providing highly specialised services, has recently been opened. However, the operations of the latter are still at very rudimentary stages.

Botswana provides universal health care to all citizens through the public health care system by operating 98% of the health facilities. However, privately run health care is also available and accessed by a privileged few with their resources [10].

The primary care model is the foundation of Botswana's healthcare system. Primary healthcare is the most economical way of achieving universal health coverage. Comprehensive care is offered throughout the lifespan and should include preventive, curative, and promotional health services [11].

The clinics primarily provide outpatient services within reach of communities, including general consultations, health prevention, and promotion services. Health posts offer limited services, whereas mobile stops need a permanent structure and are serviced by clinics and health posts within their catchment area. In the lowest-level facilities are health posts run by at least two general nurses and a health care assistant or a health education officer.

This extensive network of health facilities is well integrated to complement preventive, promotive, and rehabilitative health services and treatment and care of common health problems for citizens [11]. Primary health care services include immunisations, maternity care, children's health, prevention of communicable diseases, environmental health, nutrition, school health services, first aid, drug education, accident prevention, emergency services, and assistance with family life education [9]. In addition, health Education Assistants conduct health promotion activities by providing basic healthcare advice and health education materials to families and communities [12].

Botswana's healthcare system advocates for community participation in health promotion and prevention. Community involvement through community leaders and support groups to improve health promotion and prevention. The support groups' mission is to work with expectant mothers before and after pregnancy, expectant mothers who are HIV-positive pregnant, teenagers, and underage children engaging in sexual activity. There are discussion groups known as "Botsogo Pitso", a different approach aiming to promote interaction with patients and the communities, inform them of the services provided, and solicit their feedback.

These different health strategies and approaches have greatly influenced the improvement of health indicators and access. However, all the country's health concerns have not been alleviated because, like many countries in Sub-Saharan Africa, Botswana is still battling high rates of HIV and AIDS, other infectious diseases and currently with an upsurge of non-communicable diseases.

3.2 Traditional health care

The traditional healthcare system operates on beliefs, values and cultural doctrines. According to traditional Tswana philosophy, illness, death and misfortunes are never accepted as natural occurrences. Instead, they are attributed to the supernatural intervention of external agents such as ancestral spirits, supreme God powers, and sorcerers [13]. Ancestral spirits are regarded as the guardians of familial and tribal morality. They can sanction punishment for deviation from or violating familial and tribal norms with illness and misfortune [13]. Further, the supreme God, the creator of the universe and controller of everything, can inflict punishment on people by sending famine, diseases and death [13]. Lastly, the sorcerers cause illnesses and misfortune through witchcraft and manipulation of roots and herbs so that illness, death and misfortune would befall an individual [13].

Therefore, treatment interventions for people who hold these beliefs will depend on what is believed to have caused it. For example, if the illness is believed to be caused by ancestral spirits, certain rituals, such as prayers or offerings, are held to appease the spirits. If the illness is believed to be caused by sorcerers, traditional healers will be consulted to counteract the sorcery. Various traditional healers use different treatment modalities and approaches to counteract acts of sorcery. The beliefs also determine the health prevention modalities and interventions that will be instituted.

The Botswana health care system has utilised the Primary Health Care (PHC) approach to undergird its health programmes, strategies and interventions. This approach was the most feasible, realistic and relevant for an emerging nation with meagre resources and health infrastructure.

4. Primary health care strategy

PHC is viewed as an essential function in driving the country's development. As early as the 1980s, PHC was given priority in terms of funds allocation in the national

DOI: http://dx.doi.org/10.5772/intechopen.111974

development budgets, indicating the country's commitment to health care for all citizens [14].

Central to PHC are the concepts such as community participation, universal coverage and accessibility, appropriate technologies, inter-sectoral collaboration, appropriate, timely referrals and the use of community-based healthcare providers. While all concepts are essential, community participation is deemed a very critical strategy in PHC, where individuals and members of the communities assume the responsibility of improving and maintaining their health [14].

Primary Health Care is considered essential healthcare at the operational level. It includes education on current health issues and related preventive and control strategies, promotion of supply of food and appropriate nutrition, provision of safe water and basic sanitation, maternal and child healthcare, immunisations against major communicable diseases, prevention, and control of locally endemic diseases, appropriate treatment of common diseases, and provision of essential drugs.

Primary Health Care service delivery has changed due to the recent increase in non-communicable diseases in Botswana. These services are now part of the entire hospital and healthcare services range. These organisations offer treatment services for common illnesses as well as preventive, promotional, and rehabilitative health services [15].

The Ministry of Health in Botswana further adopted the World Health Organisation's package of essential non-communicable diseases (WHO PEN) recommended for low-resource settings to integrate non-communicable diseases (NCDs) into PHC [16]. The recommendations guided the development of the Botswana Primary Care Guidelines (BPCG), which the country implemented in 2017 to strengthen health promotion initiatives. The guidelines seek to aid healthcare professionals in identifying signs and symptoms of common illnesses and their management. In addition to evidence-based treatment decision support for healthcare providers, the guidelines emphasise the promotion of patient self-management through individual counselling by a nurse and a dietitian, as well as group health education, defaulter tracing and strengthening coordination of care [16].

Like other African countries, Botswana has endured increasing demands on the health care system. There have been great success stories in some areas, especially the battle against HIV and AIDS. However, despite the country's high middle-income status, Botswana has not been as successful in other areas, such as childhood malnutrition and infant and maternal mortality [17].

4.1 Health promotion processes and strategies

Botswana as a member of the World Health Organisation (WHO), was part of the Ottawa Chatter Conference (1986) agreement whose primary purpose was to enhance the health and well-being of the public [18]. The Ottawa Chatter Conference demanded that the WHO member states orchestrate five main strategies: build public policy; create supportive environments; Strengthen community action; develop personal skills and reorient health services.

Since the inception and adoption of the Ottawa Chatter agreements, Botswana has put processes and strategies in place that are geared towards attaining its vision. At the top of the strategy is the Ministry of Health MOH), whose function oversees the country's health needs, mainly through public health [19]. The mission of MOH is to "provide integrated, holistic, and sustainable preventative, curative and rehabilitative quality services in the country." MOH has eight departments: Cooperate services, clinical services, public health, HIV and AIDS prevention and care regulatory services, Health policy development monitoring and evaluation and Health hub.

The Department of Public Health provides health prevention and promotion initiatives in Botswana under Child Health, Health Promotion and Education, Sexual and Reproductive Health, Disease and Control, Environmental and Occupational Health, Nutrition and Food Control, Rehabilitation and Mental Health, Oral Health, Alcohol and Substance Abuse and Prevention of Blindness Units.

To promote health and achieve the Ottawa Chatter mandate, Botswana, through the lead of the MOH, has adopted international strategic goals such as Millennium Development Goals and the United Nations Sustainable Development Goals (SDGs) (2015). In 2000 Botswana government signed the United Nations Millennium Development Goals (MDGs), which mandated the UN member states to commit to eight goals: to combat poverty, hunger, disease, illiteracy, environmental degradation, and discrimination against women by 2015. However, the MDGs have been superseded by The United Nations Sustainable Development Goals (SDGs), which envisioned a world free of poverty, hunger, and disease. The main emphasis is on SDG3, which prompts countries to promote member states' health by 2030. In addition, health promotion initiatives recognise that social determinants of health go beyond the health sector.

In response to these strategies in 2010, the Botswana government, through the help of the American Centre for Disease, developed the "The Essential Health Service Package for Botswana, [20]. The EHSP is a set of health interventions that are promotive, preventive and curative, and rehabilitative that should be available to the entire population of the country." The essence of EHSP is that essential health care should be cost-effective, accessible and readily available to people. Furthermore, the provision of care through the EHSP is based on the ethical principles of need, cost-effectiveness and human dignity. Therefore, it is integral that health care is provided within an integrated area where public members can access care within one area rather than through a fragmented piecemeal.

The goals of the EHSP in Botswana were to ensure that all Botswana people have universal coverage of essential health care services. Accordingly, a revised National Health Policy was launched in 2011 [21] to guide the implementation. The policy strives to provide an environment where everyone in Botswana can achieve and maintain the highest health and well-being. The policy operates through the guidance of guiding principles as per **Table 1**.

4.2 Health promotion strategies in Botswana

Throughout the years, the Ministry of Health, through the Public Health Department, has made a concerted effort to develop and implement health promotion activities across the lifespan and to respond to the SDGs. These efforts incorporated strategies that promote health and well-being from childbirth across a life span. They include:

4.2.1 Early childhood

Strategies intended to promote childhood health include under-five feeding, childhood immunisation and expanded programmes on immunisation, and school health programme.

Guiding Principle	Description
Ethics	Respect for human dignity, rights, confidentiality and cultural beliefs.
Norms and Standards	Good management practices and quality assurance in service delivery.
Equity	Equitable distribution of resources to guarantee accessibility to quality services at every point of demand, especially for the vulnerable, marginalised and underserved, irrespective of political, ethnic or religious affiliations and place of domicile.
Ownership	Involvement/participation of all stakeholders (providers and users) of health services in defining policy as well as the implementation framework.
Evidence-based	The policy will be based on evidence, particularly about Botswana.
Innovation	Continuous exploration of new ideas in health care delivery, e.g. geographical targeting, to benefit high-priority areas; health insurance coverage for the disadvantaged sections of society; public-private partnership; demand-side financing; etc.
Gender Equity	Addressing gender-sensitive and responsive issues, including the equal involvement of men and women in decision-making, eliminating obstacles (barriers) to services utilisation, and the prevention of gender-based violence.
Client Satisfaction	Ensuring efficient 24-hour quality health services that are more responsive and sensitive to Customer needs.
Skilled staff retention and circulation	Attractive service conditions (package) and job satisfaction encourage a net inflow of critically required skills.
Partnerships	Increasing community empowerment; active involvement of the private sector, NGOs, local government authorities and civil society, and effective development partner coordination.

***Adopted from The guiding principles/values of the Botswana Health Policy Ministry of Health 2011.*

Table 1.
Guiding principles of the Botswana National Health Policy.

4.3 Under five feeding and immunisation programme

Botswana has put strategies in place to promote the health of children. The strategies include monitoring children's growth through local clinics and mobile stops nationwide. The services are offered by healthcare assistants under the guidance and supervision of the nurses. In addition, Botswana has a strong Integrated Management of Childhood Disorders (IMCI) programme that is implemented through the Child Health Care Division. Its aim is to reduce infant and children's mortality and promote development [22]. To achieve this, all the under-five children are expected to attend the clinics and are provided with monthly feeds under the feeding policy of the under-five. In addition, every child under five attends the child warfare clinics and receives free scheduled childhood immunisations. Furthermore, all those attending the clinic receive a package of essential feeds.

4.3.1 School health

The children enter primary education from 6 to 13 years, followed by secondary education from 14 to 17 years. The health promotion activities for these age groups are provided in schools and coordinated by the District Health Management Teams throughout the country under the National School Health Policy and Manual of 1999, whose mandate is to promote the health and well-being of school-going children in Botswana. Botswana's significant school health providers are mainly nurses of different nursing specialities.

4.3.2 Adolescent health

Most adolescent health promotion activities are provided through Youth Friendly Clinics nationwide. These clinics' mandate is to provide young people with free, confidential and barrier-free health services without intimidation. Some of the services provided include health education and counselling on adolescents' sexuality and reproductive health, living positively with HIV and other health-related issues such as information on substance abuse, mental health and prevention of rape and HIV prevention, including information on access to post-exposure prophylaxis, in case of rape. [23].

5. Young adults and older adulthood

The safe motherhood initiative framework was adopted, and it is used to ensure the safe health of childbearing families. The six pillars of the initiative include family planning, antenatal care, obstetric care, post-natal care, post-abortion care and control of sexually transmitted diseases. In addition, the country has invested in several programs as part of the global strategy for women, children and adolescent's health strategy (2016–2030), as a way to improve the health and well-being of people, including the involvement of males [24] National Guidelines on Health Services Integration.

5.1 Disease prevention and health promotion

The MOH utilises the strategic plan approach, a problem-solving strategy, to identify problems and map out possible solutions. The strategies are applied at all levels of implementation by healthcare workers under the MOH, and the reviews are quarterly to assess the progress and measure the impact of the action. The following health promotion disease prevention strategies are directed at controlling both non-communicable and communicable diseases are discussed:

6. Disease surveillance and prevention

Ministry of Health & Wellness Multi-Sectoral Strategy for the Prevention and Control of Non-Communicable Diseases 2018–2023 identified four priority areas: (a) prevention and health promotion, (b) diagnosis and treatment, and (c) monitoring, surveillance, and research. The fourth priority area, governance and coordination, requires strengthening and is critical to accelerating national NCD prevention and control efforts. In addition, reduce risk factors through awareness, promoting healthy lifestyles and creating enabling environments to create a legislative and policy [16].

The Centres for Disease Control and Prevention (CDC) established an office in Botswana in 1995 to strengthen tuberculosis prevention and control. In 2000 HIV prevention, treatment, and strategic information program development was incorporated to combat the HIV epidemic. CDC collaborates with the Botswana Ministry of Health and Wellness (MOHW), providing technical assistance and research to support HIV and TB control programs, injury prevention, and emergency response operation (https://www.cdc.gov/globalhealth/countries/botswana/). Botswana has made significant progress in adopting the Integrated Disease Surveillance and Response (IDSR) guidelines to facilitate surveillance and timely response to disease outbreaks. The experiences in managing HIV and other disease outbreaks were used to control and manage COVID-19 [17].

6.1 Non-communicable diseases

Botswana faces a transition in disease patterns shown by a decline in infectious diseases and an increase in chronic non-communicable diseases and their associated risk factors [25]. There are four major Non-Communicable Diseases (NCDs) which include cardiovascular, diabetes, cancer and chronic respiratory diseases, which account for NCDs-related morbidity and mortality in the population [16].

Cardiovascular diseases are estimated to cause 18% of mortality in the country [16]. Cardiovascular is responsible for repeat outpatient visits in both government and private facilities in Botswana. With the changing lifestyle and screening, more disease cases are diagnosed and managed. Another condition that is on the rise is diabetes mellitus which is estimated to cause 6% of all deaths in Botswana. Diabetes is the main cause of avoidable blindness leading to diabetic retinopathy. Chronic respiratory disease contributes to 4% of all deaths, while Asthma is one of the significant causes of childhood morbidity. Cancer disorders are rising, accounting for 7% of cancers in adults and children [17].

Prevention and management of diabetes are the responsibilities of the government through the Ministry of Health. All clinics in the various districts provide screening, education and management support to diabetic patients. In addition, private clinics and hospitals also provide services to some clients through government aid or individual medical insurance. The community collaborates with the government through the Diabetes Association of Botswana [24]. The main goal is to conduct support groups providing medical devices and health promotion activities. One clinic in the capital city has been designated for management of clients with diabetes. The clinic receives referrals from other parts of the country.

Improving Cancer Care and Prevention in Botswana was intensified in 2019. As a result, the five **critical** domains of care were identified: (1) Enhance workforce capacity in cancer and other NCDs involving personnel training, (2) Improve the supply of drugs and secure funds to avoid drug and equipment failure, (3) Build a standard of practice in oncology practice guidelines and Create policies that protect the public, for example, Smoke-free policies and HPV vaccinations. (4) Improve prevention education, screenings, and diagnostics in ambulatory settings, and (5) Establish screening guidelines for common cancers, such as HPV vaccination programs and breast cancer screening [18].

Primary prevention uses both community and facility as antenatal services, child welfare clinics, and vaccinations (e.g., HPV, hepatitis B). Clinics and community-based HPV), as well as enhancing awareness, advocacy, and community buy-in of the preventive services available at health facilities (e.g., hepatitis B vaccination and various types of screening).

HIV introduces excess risk to NCDs, such as cardiovascular diseases and cancers. Thus, treating HIV is also an effective strategy for preventing some NCDs [24].

Primary prevention interventions entail early detection through screening clients in health facilities and the community. Then, treatment starts for all eligible as well as care, and support is given through several structures such as home-based care programmes, hospice and community support.

6.2 Communicable diseases

6.2.1 Tuberculosis

Tuberculosis (TB) is a communicable disease that is a major cause of ill health and one of the leading causes of death worldwide [26]. In Botswana, the incidence of TB is 235/100000, including also occurring as HIV/TB comorbidities. In addition, some patients develop Multi-Drug Resistant (MDR) infections with about 15/1000. Low-income populations with poor housing are mostly affected.

The Ministry of Health in Botswana established the National Tuberculosis Programme (BNTP) in 1975 to fight the spread of tuberculosis. A community-based care approach that reaches patients in the community was established [26]. The country adopted the Centres for Disease Control and Prevention (CDC) 1995 treatment strategy focused on tuberculosis and HIV prevention. In addition, the African Comprehensive HIV/AIDS Partnerships (ACHAP) contributes to eradicating the diseases in line with the WHO and the United Nations (UN) Member States' strategy. The effort focuses on preventative treatment, poverty alleviation and research to reduce the infection rate by 90% in 2035 [26]. As a result, the treatment success rate is high, including in patients with HIV on treatment [27].

6.2.2 Human immunodeficiency virus (HIV)

The HIV infection is monitored and evaluated using Surveys. The (BAIS V) conducted in 2021 revealed an annual incidence of HIV among adults aged 15–64 years in Botswana was 0.2%, which is 2200 new cases of HIV per year among adults. HIV incidence was 0.4% among females and 0.0% among males [28]. Females are the most affected, with a prevalence of 26.2 and 15.2% among males. HIV infection among children aged 0–14 in Botswana was 0.8%. That is 5600 children living with HIV. The study revealed high viral Load suppression among adults aged 15–64 years living with HIV in Botswana [29]. Botswana has greatly succeeded in combating the infection, and now the country strives for zero infection.

6.2.3 Malaria

Malaria cases are mainly found in six districts in the northern-most part of Botswana: Bobirwa, Boteti, Chobe, Ngamiland, Okavango, and Tutume. However, some cases were reported in the district in the central-eastern part of the country due to increased rainfall and stagnant water in those areas. A national team leads the control and elimination strategies for malaria. Malaria cases are estimated at 0.6/100000 by 2021 [30].

6.2.4 COVID-19

Clients with acute respiratory symptoms are screened and tested for COVID-19. Supportive care is given to patients who test positive for COVID-19. The infection is classified under notifiable diseases, recorded and reported daily to the COVID-19 task team. An average number of cases is computed every 7 days. The incidence is 19 cases per million people in 2023 [17]. The Ministry of Health controls the spread of infection in partnership with the Centre for Disease Control (CDC). The CDC coordinates the activities regarding; surveillance, diagnoses and capacity building, quarantine, case investigation, infection prevention and control [31]. The fight against the epidemic was a success because the experiences and capacity used in managing other public health problems that occurred in the past were used to conduct health prevention strategies such as quarantine, disease surveillance and case management.

7. Maternal and child illnesses

Most women (97.2%) attend Antenatal Care (ANC) and deliver in hospitals under the care of midwives and doctors. However, maternal mortality continues to be a concern, with an increase in Maternal Mortality Ratio (MMR) of 166.7/100000 live births in 2019 [32]. The deaths of women are attributable to haemorrhage (28%), puerperal sepsis (24.7%) and hypertension (17%). Nonetheless, the infant mortality rate is declining. Botswana's infant mortality rate in 2023 is 26.744 deaths per 1000 live births.

7.1 National campaigns

The MOHW conducts health campaigns annually to respond to the country's health needs. They mainly include under-five polio and measles campaigns, where children are given vaccines depending on their needs. There are also malaria campaigns in wet areas of the country. The Public Health and Environmental Health Department, under the Ministry of Health's leadership, plays a significant role in preventing and controlling malaria throughout the country [33].

7.2 Health education strategies

The Health Education Unit is critical in facilitating the country's health information, education and communication campaigns. Health educators and nurses lead in educating the communities on public health issues. In addition, different media platforms, such as the National Television and Radio, and social media are used [34].

7.3 Challenges

Botswana is trying to meet the SDGs and Ottawa Chatter agreements, but some things must be fixed [25]. For example, the country needs more healthcare personnel to implement health promotion initiatives. There is also a need for more resources such as funds, human capital, infrastructural development and transport to render other areas of the country accessible to basic amnesties.

8. Conclusion

This chapter has discussed health promotion and disease prevention in Botswana. It situated health promotion within Botswana by outlining the health care system.

It described primary health care as the main framework on which health promotion and services are based. Further, the health promotion strategies, approaches, programmes, and interventions that promote health promotion were discussed. These are approaches that promote early childhood, immunisation programmes, care of the under-fives and immunisations, school health disease surveillance and disease prevention, health campaigns and health education strategies. Health promotion and disease prevention are very critical in any healthcare setting. Not only do health promotion strategies ensure equitable resource distribution, but they also guarantee access to health care delivery. Finally, this chapter has illustrated the implementation of health promotion in Botswana. It concluded by outlining the processes, strategies, health programmes and approaches that have been put in place for its implementation.

Author details

Esther Salang Seloilwe*, Kebope Mongie Kealeboga, Joyce V. Khutjwe, Lesedi Mosebetsi and Tebogo T. Mamalelala
School of Nursing, University of Botswana, Gaborone, Botswana

*Address all correspondence to: seloilwe@ub.ac.bw

References

[1] World Health Organization World Health Organization. The 1st International Conference on Health Promotion, Ottawa, 1986. 2023. Available from: https://www.who.int/teams/health-promotion/enhanced-wellbeing/first-global-conference. [Accessed: May 22, 2023]

[2] United States of America Center for Disease Control and Prevention. Data Collection Methods for Evaluation: Document Review. 2018. Available from: https://www.cdc.gov/healthyyouth/evaluation/pdf/brief18.pdf [Acessed June 22, 2023]

[3] Ministry of Health. Annual Report, Government Printers, Gaborone. 1979

[4] Ministry of Health of Health web page. Available from: www.gov.bw [Accessed: April 11, 2023]

[5] Statistics Botswana web page. Available from: www.statsbots.org.bw. [Accessed: April 11, 2023]

[6] Health and Nutrition. Available from: www.unicef.org. [Accessed: April, 2023]

[7] Ministry of Finance. Botswana National Development plans, 10,11. 2023. Available from: https://www.finance.gov.bw/index.php?option=com_content&view=category&id=28&Itemid=126 [Accessed may 22, 2023]

[8] Seloilwe ES, Thupayagale-Tshweneagae G. Community mental health care in Botswana: Approaches and opportunities. International Nursing Review. 2007;**54**:173-178. DOI: 10.1111/j.1466-7657.2007.00525.x [Accessed June 2023]

[9] Ministry of Health. Available from: www.org.bw. [Accessed: May, 2023]

[10] Walshe K, Smith J. Health Care Management. 3rd ed. London: Open University Press; 2016

[11] Nkomazana O. A Healthcare Case Study from Botswana, Africa. Springer International Publishing; EBooks. Springer Nature. 2022. DOI: 10.1007/978-3-030-68458-7_23. [Accessed May 02, 2023]

[12] Tapela NM, Tshisimogo G, Shatera BP, Letsatsi V, Gaborone M, Madidimalo T, et al. Integrating non-communicable disease services into primary health care, Botswana. Bulletin of the World Health Organization. 2019;**97**(2):142-153. DOI: 10.2471/BLT.18.221424 Epub 2019 08 January

[13] Kupe SS. An Uneasy Walk to Quality: The Evolution of Black Nursing Education. Battle Creek: Michigan: W.K Kellogg Foundation; 1993

[14] Tapera R, Moseki S, January J. The status of health promotion in Botswana. Journal of public health in Africa. 2018;**9**(1):699. DOI: 10.4081/jphia.2018.699

[15] Botswana Population Census 2022. Statistics Botswana. Available from: www.statsbots.org.bw. [Accessed: April, 2023]

[16] Ministry of Health. Botswana Multi–Sectoral Strategy for the Prevention and Control of Non-Communicable Diseases 2018-2023. Republic of Botswana: Ministry of Health; 2018. pp. 1-48

[17] Centre for Disease Control and Prevention. CDC in Botswana. 2023;**201**. Available from: https://www.cdc.gov/globalhealth/countries/botswana/default.htm. [Accessed April 11, 2023]

[18] Ministry of Health. Improving Cancer Care and Prevention in Botswana: Workshop Report August 7th –8th 2019 Gaborone. Ministry of Health. 2919. Available from: https://globalhealth.rutgers.edu/wp-content/uploads/botswana-cancer-care-and-prevention-workshop-report.pdf [Accessed: May 02, 2023]

[19] World Health Organization. Health Promotion Emblem. 2023. Available from: https://www.who.int/teams/health-promotion/enhanced-wellbeing/first-global-conference/emblem [Accessed May 02, 2023]

[20] MoHW. Extended Malaria Strategic Plan 2014-2018: Towards Malaria Elimination National Malaria Programme. Gaborone: MoHW; 2014

[21] Ministry of Health. The essential health package for Botswana. 2010. Available from: https://www.moh.gov.bw/Publications/policies/Botswana%20EHSP%20HLSP.pdf. [Accessed: May 2, 2023]

[22] Ministry of Health. Departments & Programs. 2023. Available from: https://www.moh.gov.bw/about_us_departments.html. [Accessed: May 2, 2023]

[23] Tjirare LT, Tlale J. Improving child health care in Botswana: What can be done? The Pan African Journal. 2021;**39**:242. DOI: 10.11604/pamj.2021.39.242.29139

[24] WHO. Global tuberculosis report 2021. Contract No. Available from: https://github.com/hazimtimimi/tb_profiles

[25] Fiscal year. Available from: https://www.unicef.org/esa/media/5461/file/UNICEF-Botswana-2019-Health-Budget-Brief.pdf.

[26] Siamisang K, Rankgoane-Pono G, Madisa TM, Mudiayi T, Tlhakanelo JT. Outcomes, and predictors of tuberculosis mortality in Kweneng West District, Botswana: A retrospective cohort study. The Pan African Medical Journal. 2022;**2022**(42):1

[27] Statistics Botswana. Botswana Fifth AIDS Impact Survey (BAIS IV) 2022. Report. Statistics Botswana. Available from: https://www.statsbots.org.bw/sites/default/files/BAIS%20V%20Preliminary%20Report.pdf [Accessed May 02, 2023]

[28] Onen BL, Harris C, Ignatowicz A, Davies J, Drouvelis M, Howes A, et al. Ageing, frailty and resilience in Botswana: Rapid ageing, rapid change. Findings from a national working group meeting and literature review. BMC Proceedings. 2019;**13**(Suppl. 10):8

[29] Keetile M, Navaneetham K, Letamo G, Rakgoasi SD. Socioeconomic inequalities in non-communicable disease risk factors in Botswana: A cross-sectional study. BMC Public Health. 2019;**19**(1):1060

[30] Statistics Botswana. Botswana Maternal Mortality Ratio. 2019 Report. Statistics Botswana. 2019. Available from: https://www.statsbots.org.bw/sites/default/files/publications/Botswana%20Maternal%20Mortality%20Ratio%20%202019.pdf [Accessed April 11, 2023]

[31] Centre for Disease Control and Prevention. Division of Global Health and Protection. Collaborating to Strengthen Surveillance Systems Worldwide. 2023. Available from: https://www.cdc.gov/globalhealth/healthprotection/fieldupdates/2022/Collaborating-to-Strengthen-Surveillance-Systems-Worldwide.html#:~:text=CDC%20is%20

collaborating%20with%20countries,timely%2C%20complete%2C%20and%20representative. [Accessed: May 12, 2023]

[32] Ministry of Health. National Health Policy "Towards a Healthier Botswana." 2011. Available from: https://www.moh.gov.bw/Publications/policies/revised_National_Health_Policy.pdf. [Accessed: May 2, 2023]

[33] UNFPA. How to Establish a Youth Friendly: tips for star YFS performance. 2016. Available from: https://botswana.unfpa.org/sites/default/files/pub-pdf/wallchartA3.pdfUNFP. [Accessed: May 2, 2023]

[34] Ministry of Health. NATIONAL GUIDELINES ON HEALTH SERVICES INTEGRATION Reproductive, Maternal, Newborn, Child, and Adolescent, Health, Nutrition, Non-Communicable Diseases & Other Services. 2021. Available from: https://esaro.unfpa.org/sites/default/files/pub-pdf/botswana_national_guidelines_report_v2_for_printing_18.05.22_1.pdf. [Accessed: May 2, 2023]